MW01166582

Blessed Assurance
Success Despite the Odds

"I endorse [Blessed Assurance: Success Despite the Odds] and readily commend it to both professional and lay audiences. It is, at once, inspiring and instructive—infusing ample doses of love and humor."

Rev. Dr. Percy L. Moore
Retired Professor, Wayne State University

"What an amazing testimony. Her story will inspire others to remain strong and keep faith amid life's many whirlwind encounters."

Rev. Dr. Carlyle Fielding Stewart, III
Sr. Pastor, Hope United Methodist Church

"Blessed Assurance: Success Despite the Odds was really an inspiration to me. I started reading it on the plane and could not put it down."

Emma Oliver
President, Hope United Methodist Women

Blessed Assurance

Success Despite the Odds

By Jacquie Lewis-Kemp

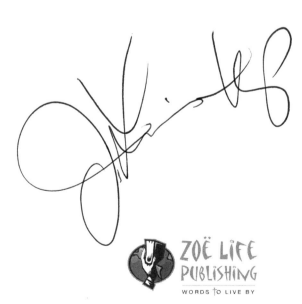

ZOË LIFE
PUBLISHING
WORDS TO LIVE BY

Published by:
Zoë Life Publishing
P.O. Box 871066
Canton, MI 48187 USA
www.zoelifepub.com

Author: Jacqueline Lewis-Kemp
Cover Design: Jamie Anipen
Editorial Team: Denise Crittendon and Bethany Savage

First U.S. Edition 2009

Publisher's Cataloging-In-Publication Data

Lewis-Kemp, Jacqueline

Blessed Assurance

Summary: Story about overcoming despite life's obstacles, including, diabetes, West Nile virus, a double organ transplant and death of loved ones.

10 Digit ISBN 1-934363-63-4 Soft Cover, Perfect Bind
13 Digit ISBN 978-1-934363-63-8 Soft Cover, Perfect Bind

      1.   Juvenile diabetes, Business, Success, Inspirational, Transplant-Pancreas, Transplant-Kidney, Christian Living, Automotive Industry, Chronic Illness, Balance of work and family

Library of Congress Control Number: 2009928475

For current information about releases by Jacqueline Lewis-Kemp or other releases from Zoë Life Publishing, visit our website: http://www.zoelifepub.com

Printed in the United States of America

V8.1 10 16 09

In Loving Memory

In Memory of my parents
Jim and Jean Lewis

"Blessed assurance, Jesus is mine
Oh what a foretaste of glory divine
Heir of salvation, purchase of God
Born of His spirit, washed in his blood
This is my story, this is my song
Praising my Savior all the daylong"

Fanny J. Crosby, 1873

Acknowledgements

Writing this book has forced me to look at my life in much more detail than my daily pulse of how I feel about my life so far. I have always known that I am blessed and that God has brought me through some seemingly impossible circumstances. But my God is so much more than just a 911 God who shows up when I'm in trouble. His power and might is evident in the pages that follow. I want to thank God for postponing my book writing, because I had no idea what I'd write about. I thank God for giving me something to write about. Beyond the book, I want to thank Him for the relationship with Him I've grown to understand and build my life upon.

I also want to thank my family for being so understanding as I searched to find purpose in my life after Lewis Metal Stamping—my husband and son most especially. I want to thank again, and to a larger audience, my brother Jeff who unselfishly walked with me through my kidney failure and ultimately gave me the gift of life—his left kidney. I want to thank his wife Alice, who could have talked her husband out of donating his kidney and reminded him of his obligation to her and their son—but she didn't, instead she supported both of us. Similarly, I'd like to thank the family that made the courageous decision to donate the pancreas I received to end my dependence on insulin injections and better preserve my new kidney.

I will forever be indebted to the skilled hands and minds of the University of Michigan Transplant Team and most especially my dear friend Richard Chenault. It is clear that

Christ placed Richard in my life and the lives of many to make life on earth a better place. God called Richard and five other members of the transplant team home when the Survival Flight plane crashed while leaving Milwaukee with life saving organs on its way home to Ann Arbor.

Finally, I want to thank people who helped me publish this book such as Roy Collins, III, Pam Perry at Ministry Marketing Solutions and Sabrina Adams and everyone at Zoe Life Publishing. Also critical in encouraging me were my sisters in Christ—the Divas in Milwaukee and Detroit, whose constant support on the e-line for writing this book kept me going. With the amount of prayer, support and laughter between us via the Internet, God is not only awesome, but technologically able.

Blessed Assurance

Success Despite the Odds

By Jacquie Lewis-Kemp

Table of Contents

Forward

The observation, study and practice of building and running a business have been my personal fascination for near 55 of my 60 years of life. I was born to a hard scrabble shopkeeper and rum store operator in Kingston, Jamaica, worked in and around Fortune 50 companies in the USA, both as practitioner and consultant and currently I run a manufacturer of industrial products in Mexico and the US. Jacquie is, in my view, delightfully unique and a rare find in this generally corporate world of sameness. She is courageous, funny and delightful all at the same time. This book provides glimpses where these qualities are on display constantly.

Taking over and developing Lewis Metal after her beloved father's passing was indeed courageous. There was a myriad of reasons to do otherwise—cut and run comes to mind immediately—since the obstacles were so large and seemingly insurmountable. I entered Jacquie's sphere around this period and watched with great affection, admiration and awe as she did battle with some of the corporate clones that seem to exist only to discourage enterprise and initiative, which she had in great abundance. The work was often frustrating at times, but had great promise for folks like Jacquie who was willing to roll up her sleeves and challenge the orthodoxy of the day. Young black women did not belong in the rough and tumble world of automotive supply. Despite the lack of great financial results that eluded her because of capital access, Jacquie persevered and triumphed, demonstrating that she had the acumen, sensitivity and energy to compete.

Jacquie's delightful and funny personality however is

best demonstrated in her roles as mother, wife, daughter, sister and general family glue while functioning as business leader. I was diagnosed with diabetes 2 to 3 years earlier. Jacquie became my personal and unpaid advisor to life in this bewildering world of diabetes management. She helped me make sense of the medical pronouncements from my doctors, translating them into everyday practical dos and don'ts. As one would imagine my schedule was hectic by living and working from homes and offices in California and Ohio. It was her thoughtful, insistent advice that helped my self-management of this all too prevalent disease. This book will share these insights with a wider audience and all will be enriched by reading and sharing her story, as my family and I were as we watched it unfold.

Francis L. Price,
President and CEO, Q3 Industries

Introduction

I developed a severe case of the West Nile virus the year that Michigan saw 450 cases. I was among the 50 that survived. However the month long hospital stay left me unable to walk unassisted, with severe speech impediment and no memory of what happened in the hospital. A little more than a year after my battle with the West Nile virus, a dear friend of my mother's offered me a position in his company. I definitely wanted to return to work, not just because we needed the money—and we did, but to exercise my brain.

Even though I wanted to return to work, that didn't necessarily mean I was ready to return. Physically, I wasn't ready. I probably wasn't ready to begin driving since I still suffered from dizziness whenever I diverted my attention. The dizziness made it difficult for me to check rear view mirrors and then return my attention to the traffic in front of me. Walking and turning corners in the office was difficult as well. Since the dizziness worsened at intersections when I had to look both ways and time traffic, I made every attempt to turn at lights so that traffic would stop as I turned. I did my best to avoid intersections without traffic lights and situations I knew would make me dizzy.

The stint of my West Nile illness that prevented me from working created a financial hardship for our family. However, working for nearly a year allowed us to rebuild our reserves and smooth out our cash flow. After trying to sell our house for the previous four years, and being stopped by my illnesses, we finally managed to move at what turned out to be timing that maximized our home's value—the perfect time to sell.

Working was tough. The job requirements were actually quite easy. However, the physical requirement of getting to and from work and moving about was difficult. In fact, in the winter I slipped and fell while trying to enter the building. The fall itself didn't hurt, but knowing that I couldn't recover from a simple imbalance on ice confirmed that I had not fully recovered and that it could be years until I was back to my old self.

I began to feel sorry for myself and began to think backwards to identify what the true culprit of my challenges was. I contracted West Nile and suffered such a severe case of it because I was immunosuppressed. Some people got the virus and barely had cold symptoms. For me, it was debilitating. My immune system was suppressed medically in order to keep my body from fighting my transplanted kidney and pancreas. My life saving kidney transplant ended my dialysis due to kidney failure and my pancreas transplant normalized by diabetic blood sugar in order to preserve my new kidney. Ah ha! All this ultimately occurred because of my diabetes. More than 30 years of Type I or juvenile diabetes wears on the body.

But despite the battles I faced everyday in life, the one thing I have come to realize in life is with every great victory a great battle must proceed it. I am still standing, and because of God's Blessed Assurance I am here to fight another day - despite the odds.

Chapter One

Growing Up with Diabetes

Diabetes – How it All Happened

*I*t was amazing how it all happened. My maternal grandparents often took me on fishing trips. It was our chance to eat pizza and enjoy the outdoors—not to mention catch that day's dinner. We went to a place in Canada with a long dock where many people fished. My grandmother always packed for "just in case." She had extra food, a jug of water to drink and another to wash our hands. She had extra clothes for us, including shoes. She learned the importance of this after my cousin fell in the river and my grandfather saved her. Granny had a complete change of clothes for my cousin, but only had a towel for Granddaddy.

Fishing trips were so frequent that it was my grandmother

who noticed my symptoms of diabetes. We were fishing on the dock when I had to go to the bathroom really bad. My grandmother walked me back up the dock to use the public restroom. Knowing she had a jug of water, I wanted a cup of it. She obliged and we returned to the fishing spot.

No sooner than when I got back to my chair, I had to go to the bathroom again. So, my grandmother escorted me again up the dock to the public restrooms. Again, I was thirsty so my grandmother gave me more water and decided to take it out to where we were fishing so that all of us could enjoy it. Out of the entire jug, Granddaddy may have had a cup; however, I remember drinking the ice dry in the two-gallon thermos. We also made several more trips to the bathroom.

When we returned home, Granny told my mom that she'd better get me checked out by the doctor because we didn't fish a lick. And so at my two-month old baby brother's next appointment with the doctor, she asked the doctor to check me out. Without the normal diabetic test, a glucose tolerance test, they drew a random blood sugar test. My blood sugar tested very high, well out of the normal range. Mom's two-month-old son was fine, but her daughter was diabetic.

I was seven when I was diagnosed with diabetes. It was in August, 1969. My recollection of my first night at the hospital is visions of bright chrome and white porcelain. My father always told me stories at bedtime and so in the hospital he also told me one until I drifted off to sleep.

The first night I woke up after he left. I jumped from my bed and ran screaming down the halls. The nurses quieted me and put me back to bed promising that he would return in the morning. The only place I had spent the night prior to the hospital stay was at my grandparents' house.

The doctors spent time not only regulating my blood sugar, but also teaching me to manage my diabetes—the most important of which was to give myself a shot. The days in the hospital got better as they explained that I would learn to give myself shots. That sounded like I would be a doctor. Sure enough before I left the hospital, I knew how to give myself an insulin shot and my parents knew how to sterilize my glass syringe and draw up my insulin.

My grandparents also visited me in the hospital. And my grandfather, who was the pastor of our church, told me, "Not to worry, we'll pray this away." I don't recall all of the circumstances, but I remember him saying those words, and my father being uncomfortable with my grandfather's proclamation. Dad didn't want me to spend time hoping this condition would one day disappear.

Juvenile diabetes is a chronic illness and there is no cure for it. The doctors explained to my parents that the most difficult task ahead of them was to make sure I understood that I would always need to take insulin injections and follow a diabetic diet. And at the same time, they had to make sure that I understood that the diabetes wouldn't stop me from growing up to be a successful adult.

I missed two months of second grade. I couldn't wait to tell my friends that I'd been away at medical training and could give myself a shot—not just once, but every day. Back then diabetes wasn't diagnosed nearly as often as it is now and no one in my family had juvenile onset diabetes. I remember my parents reassuring me that this disease meant that I just needed to manage my health, live and eat properly. Whenever I asked, "What should I be when I grow up?" Both parents would always answer, "Whatever you want to be as long as it is something you enjoy. You can do whatever you want, as long as you work hard at it." Amazing how I still believe that 40 years later.

Managing diabetes with the best that 1970s technology had to offer was a challenge. Diabetes was managed by urine sugar because there was no home glucose monitoring system. We used Tes-Tape™, which when dipped in urine either remained yellow if you had no sugar in your urine, slightly green if you had trace amounts and darker greens for moderate to high sugar levels. It was a formidable task to pee on a 2" x ¼" strip of tape without making a mess all over your hands— and if I touched the test area, the sweat on my hands would react with the tape and cause the test to falsely read higher.

I went to diabetic camp as a child where all the children were diabetic. Before each meal we had to test our urine and report it to the counselor who then recorded it and turned it into the medical staff at camp. The doctors, nurses and dieticians used it to determine what your insulin doses should be. If you couldn't pee before a meal, you couldn't eat until you did. There is not much worse than cold camp mashed potatoes scooped out in ½ cup scoops. The camp experience was an important one. The normal camp activities proved that I could do anything while being diabetic. Being with children who were also diabetic showed me that I wasn't alone on this journey.

My doctor's appointments were every six months. My blood sugar was monitored and the doctor reviewed my log of urine sugars, food, and activity level at different times of the day. Then, based upon urine sugar trends, the doctor gave me an insulin dosage to take each day until my next visit. Insulin was different then, too. Long before the days of Humulin™, made from e-coli bacteria, there was insulin made from beef and pork pancreases. At that time there were two different strengths of insulin: U-40 and U-80. If a person took a dose of 40 units or less they bought U-40 insulin and U-40 syringes. Likewise, if a person took more than 40 units they used U-80 insulin and U-80 syringes.

To complicate matters more, before plastic disposable syringes, I was sent home from the hospital with a glass syringe that my mother sterilized each morning by boiling it. There was nothing more painful than drawing up the proper dose, assembling the disposable needle onto the syringe, and then injecting it into my thigh, only to have the residue from boiling the glass syringe cause the plunger to get stuck–while still in my thigh! No matter how hard I pushed the plunger, the insulin wouldn't go in. I'd have to withdraw it, push to check the plunger, replace the disposable needle and draw up more insulin and stick myself again.

Sometimes it wasn't the residue from the water, but the low technology of the needle. There was no such thing as microfine needles in 1969. They were longer than necessary and hurt!

Sleep overs required special consideration, too. Mom's rule was that I left my friends' house early to come home and take my insulin, and I could perhaps return if they weren't serving pancakes (which required syrup that I couldn't have) for breakfast. Because the taste of artificial sweeteners was so awful in the late '60s and '70s, I often opted to eliminate certain foods from my diet rather than ruin them with a sugarless alternative. For instance sugarless candy tasted like cough drops, so I didn't eat candy unless it had sugar and I was cheating on my diet. Sugarless syrup tasted awful too, so I didn't eat pancakes, waffles or French toast. For a long time, sugarless pop came in only two varieties cola and lemon lime. The saccharine in them forced water to taste just fine. Even as I got older, rather than use artificial sweeteners in coffee or tea, I would drink them black.

As a kid, the one thing that made life with diabetes worth living was Hog-Wild Days. My doctor allowed his diabetics to choose 3 days out of the year when we could eat anything we wanted to eat. When one of those days hit, hog-wild is what it was. I would eat pancakes with chocolate chips, ice cream and whipped cream for breakfast, candy and chips for lunch and a fast food milk shake for dinner. On these days, the doctor prescribed extra insulin and my mother monitored me closely. I always chose Halloween as one of those days so I could eat as much candy as I could (well, as much as my mother would allow), and Easter because there was always chocolate in the Easter basket for my brother. I could never get enough of the bacon the men of the church cooked after the Easter Sunday sunrise service. And, of course, I chose Christmas to enjoy all the holiday desserts.

We lived in Westland, Michigan near most of my Dad's family. My brother and I never knew a babysitter, my paternal grandmother took care of us—just like she took care of most of her grandchildren. It sometimes got confusing because we called both my grandmothers "Granny". I would distinguish them by saying, Lillian Granny when I meant my maternal grandmother; and Hattie Granny when I meant my paternal grandmother.

My dad was the youngest of seven children. Seven children gave her 28 grandchildren and 45 great-grandchildren at the time of her death. She always had a house full of people, mostly family. If not her children returning home from a divorce or to save money, it was the grandchildren who needed babysitting. Her oldest daughter was 20 years old when my grandmother was pregnant with my father. Therefore, my dad's sister and my mother's mother were the same age. I wasn't born when my paternal grandfather died of lung cancer. However, I heard lots of stories from my grandmother and Daddy. Hattie Granny's grandfather was a slave and she would often tell us stories that he told her. His gravestone now sits in the North American Black Historical Museum in Amherstburg, Ontario, where it is believed that he escaped slavery and settled. Because of that, Granny was born a Canadian citizen. Hattie Granny also told me what it was like growing up in rural Canada as a little girl. Whenever we drove to Amherstburg, I always imagined what it was like for the slaves who escaped to freedom by crossing the Detroit River by either walking across the ice or on rafts, to Canada. Hattie Granny was born in 1900 so it was always easy to remember how old she was. If it was 1976, then she was 76 years old. She became an American citizen when she married her first husband, an American. I recall her telling us that her first husband was selfish, mean and not a good provider for the family of then five children. Her first husband's name is now used as a verb in our family to describe a mean and selfish person. I reminisce now about how fortunate I am to have heard these stories first hand.

I remember a picture we once took of Hattie Granny when she was in her late 60s sitting on my brother Jeff's Big Wheel bike. Jeff asked if she would play with him and said that he wanted her to ride the Big Wheel, so she tried. It was so low to the ground that she had to wait until my dad came home to help her get off the bike. It was our family joke that Jeff could get Granny to do anything. When he was a toddler, Hattie Granny leaned her head out of the door to yell down the street for me to come in from riding my bike. Evidently I was out of earshot or didn't want to hear her. So Jeff, then a two-year-old, in an effort to be helpful, yelled, "Jacquie, Jacquie, damn you!" We still laugh about it now.

On the weekends, to get us out of the house so that my mom could clean, she sent me outside to play jacks on the front porch with my friends. My mother felt it was time for me to start taking on some responsibility so she told me to watch my three-year-old brother. I gave him the ugly Barbie™ doll to play with and continued to play jacks with my friends. Minutes later my mom looked out to check on us and didn't see her son. She asked me, "Where is Jeff?" I looked around the yard and didn't see him. We lived in a subdivision that wasn't frequently traveled, but it is still upsetting whenever a three year old is missing. My girlfriends looked just as frantic as I did and understood when I didn't take my next turn. Just then I remembered that he always liked the playground at my school, which was right around the corner, at the end of a dead end street. He always wanted to go to school with me because he thought I went to play on the playground.

So I jumped on my bike and rode around the corner in search of Jeff. The school janitor stopped me in the driveway and asked if I was looking for a boy and a dog. I told him yes, and he said, "He's that way going toward the playground." As I sped off on my bike I saw Jeff on the gravel headed for the merry-go-round on his Big Wheel with our family dog trotting along behind him. As I hoped and prayed, he was fine. He just wanted to play on the playground. After my mother was assured that Jeff was ok, she sent my friends home, and while

I braced myself for the worst punishment ever, she knew that the scare was punishment enough. Maybe that's why I'm so insistent about my own son understanding responsibility.

Our family dog, Puff, was a Pekinese who was old and protective of Jeff and me. So if you had visions of Jeff being protected by a Rottweiler, Labrador or German Shepard, that wasn't the case...at least not in Puff's physical stature. Now, if someone tried to lay a hand on Jeff, Puff would have growled, snarled and perhaps taken a bite as if he was one of those larger breeds. I'm sure Puff went along to protect Jeff. And believe me, no one could have messed with Jeff or their ankles and feet would have been eaten! Puff was a little dog with a big heart, and even bigger ego, and mean as a cuss. Puff often got into fights with other dogs and lost because he chose to fight breeds much larger than he was. Puff cost my dad a lot of money fighting. Puff had epilepsy and took medication. He had an operation on his heart from a fight and once had his eye pop out of the socket. He lost his eyesight in that eye, but the doctor was able to put it back into the socket. Of course all this happened at night after business hours, so my dad always paid emergency vet fees. Puff finally died in a fight and my dad picked him up and buried him in our yard. My mom let me miss school that morning.

We're dog people so we soon got a new Old English Sheep Dog puppy and named her Daisy. She later had five puppies. What a great experience for children to witness dogs giving birth and nurturing their young. We gave my grandmother and aunt the puppy we liked most, Butch. She lived about three miles from our house, separated by some pretty major streets. Daisy's puppy, Butch, missed his mom so much and was so sick of my aunt yelling at him that he ventured out to find his mama, Daisy. One day after my grandmother reported that he was missing, my mother looked out of the kitchen window and saw Butch in the neighbor's yard barking and licking Daisy through the fence.

We brought Butch into our yard and let the dogs visit for awhile. I wanted to keep Butch but my dad said he was Hattie Granny's dog now and we don't need two dogs. So back he went; but not for long. Butch ventured out again, but this time he wasn't so fortunate. My dad drove the route from my grandmother's house to our house and found him on the side of a major street. We mourned the loss and wondered if somehow Daisy knew.

I didn't realize until I was an adult that pets provide children with so much more than entertainment, but also friendship, protection and a sense of responsibility. A dog's life usually spans about 12-15 years. There are cases of dogs or cats living longer, but it is typically much shorter than the human life span. So kids get to experience all that happens to a pet and how it affects the family. It was important for me because in the case of our animals, I learned lots of life lessons. Our animals had litters of puppies and kittens, and so I saw the miracle of birth. And when they died, I experienced the grief and loss that death brings. While it was the loss of an animal and not a person or close family member, the feeling of loss sort of worked like antibodies. Once inoculated with grief from the loss of a pet, when death happened again, although at an increased level of grief, I recall that the pain lessened as I learned to make adjustments for life without the loved one. I understood that even though I wouldn't see them, the memory of who they were in my life would remain for ever.

Many people believe that the death of a pet is nothing

like the death of a family member. And indeed the degree of grief is much more intense when losing a family member. However, experiencing the death of a pet usually primes us or better prepares us for a much more devastating eventuality.

When I was diagnosed diabetic, my mom took an open ended leave of absence from her job. In my teenage estimation, having her home meant that she was always in my way and we no longer had as much money as we used to. My dad worked for the same company but at a different location. We occasionally had dinner with my dad's coworkers and their families. As an adult I now realize what a wonderful experience it was that we shared so much with other cultures and learned other customs. I was a kid then, and as far as I knew, everybody had friends of a different culture; had friends that didn't look like them. But what I didn't realize was that my parents were teaching me not just tolerance, but acceptance, inclusion and love for all that God made, long before I experienced the inevitable racism that I would come to know. In fact, as an adult I shared this story with a colleague and he pointed out to me that because my parents taught me appreciation for all cultures, even those who don't look like me, I tended to have naïve recognition of racism. All I knew was that I had my first girlhood crush on one of my dad's Asian Indian friend's son.

As I approached middle school, my parents grew concerned about their choice of public middle schools and knew that they wanted to move to another district. My lifelong friend Lisa lived across the street and her parents felt the same way. They always wanted lots of room and a farm. And so Mr. Smith found five acres, and talked my dad into buying five acres next door to him, and my dad talked my grandfather (my mom's dad) into buying five acres next to him. Lisa's parents and mine built homes on their property for us to move into by the time 7th grade started. Our house was legally ready to inhabit, however it was nowhere near finished. We added the finished flooring, carpet and tile, later. It was September and we had electricity, but not quite a heating system. It began to get chilly and we used space heaters until we got a heating system before November. With the expense of building a new house and Jeff entering kindergarten, Mom went back to work. She returned to work and then asked to be transferred closer to home. My dad had a main level bedroom built in our new house for his mother, Hattie Granny, to come and live with us.

Lisa and I lived next door to one another on a mile long road with four other houses on the road. Our fathers wanted the illusion of a house on a hill and so they each had ponds dug behind the houses and used the dirt to bury the at-ground-level basement, creating a hill. Jeff liked the spring pond life like tadpoles, minnows, snakes and the like. I liked it at winter to ice skate on. Jeff pretended to be a speed skater on the pond going back and forth.

In the spring the pond overflowed with rain water and the dirt roads turned to mud, often stranding us. But I wouldn't change my experience living out there for anything in the world.

At about 13 or 7th grade, my blood sugar went haywire because of changing hormone levels. I was hospitalized for a week to see if maybe I needed a different insulin dose. In the 1970s it was customary to hospitalize diabetics to adjust their insulin dose. Remember, there was no such thing as glucometers (home blood glucose testing machines) of any kind, let alone portable ones. Diabetic patients kept a log of urine sugar test results measured four times a day. The doctor would schedule appointments every six weeks and measure actual blood sugar. Based upon the trends set by the urine sugar and the fasting blood sugar taken at the visit, the doctor would adjust my insulin dose. This required quite a bit of calculating from the doctor since urine sugar values reflect blood sugar history. Therefore, understanding that the data on the urine sugar logs were a derivative of blood sugar levels and they represented an average urine sugar level based upon how long urine stayed in the bladder, determining insulin requirements were at best a guesstimate.

Also in the 1970s, U-100 insulin and U-100 syringes were developed. This was an advancement because previously there were U-40 and U-80 insulin and syringes. So this universal U-100 insulin seemed to be the best thing since sliced bread, at least for those who took 100 units or less. I don't know of anyone who took more or even close to 100 units. The other advancement was that they were completely disposable. No more boiling syringes!

The other change during that hospital visit was that the doctors said that I needed to take two shots per day. This news didn't mean that my diabetes had somehow worsened, as some non-diabetics misunderstand today. The change was due to a change in diabetes management philosophy. Doctors realized that the more insulin injections could mimic a functioning pancreas, dispensing insulin when needed and not all at once, the better they could control blood sugars. Realizing that it was impractical for diabetics to take several insulin shots, they decided on two for increased control. In my particular case, what this meant was taking my shot and eating a snack before and after school sports. Well there was no way I was giving up cheerleading so I carried the insulin, syringes and a snack to school.

I got used to managing my diabetes and remaining active. I even wrote an article while in high school for the local newspaper called Diabetes: Just An Inconvenience. At that time in my life I felt pretty proud of myself—managing my diabetes and being a regular kid and all.

My parents reached out to be educated on this dreaded disease that affected our family. We continued to take diabetes classes and learned the definition and possible causes for the condition—although there is no known or proven cause of juvenile diabetes. Unlike type 2 diabetes, or "adult onset" diabetes, as it used to be called, juvenile diabetes is not caused by lifestyle and the body's inability to make enough insulin. In the case of juvenile diabetes, the pancreas cannot produce insulin at all.

As a young child I knew what islets of Langerhan were long before today's development of islet cell transplants. Doctors were careful to educate us about long-term complications of diabetes and prevention techniques. I remember ranking the complications in order of what I believed to be the least to the most severe. I had heard that a distant cousin was diabetic, and as the old folks said, "He had it so bad that he had to have a leg amputated." As visibly handicapping as that was I figured it couldn't kill me—so that was my first choice of complications (if I had to have one). I didn't count neuropathy, because a little tingling in the hands and feet couldn't really count as a complication. Next I supposed was retinopathy, or in its extreme, blindness. While blindness too is a terrible complication, it wouldn't kill me either. I ranked kidney disease as the worse possible thing that could happen. I could live with at least one kidney. But if they both failed, I could die.

As a part of my medical regimen, the doctors monitored how much protein I was spilling in my urine. Protein molecules passing through my kidneys caused holes that further damaged the kidneys. To measure the amount of protein, doctors periodically ordered a 24-hour urinalysis. That test called for me to pee into a jug for an entire 24-hour period. When you have good working kidneys lots of urine is expelled in 24 hours—especially if you have high blood sugar with the symptoms of constant thirst and frequent urination. The nurse issues a hat (medical term for a receptacle to urinate into) with a spout and a plastic jug to store the urine in. Other diabetics and I always joked that we needed more than one jug because if our blood sugar was high we can fill that up in an hour.

The urine had to be stored in a cool place and they would prefer that you refrigerate it. In the winter that was no problem because it could be stored in the garage or outside in the snow. It was more a challenge in the summer to keep it cool and not have Jell-O taste like urine, because it shared the same space in the fridge.

My Spiritual Foundation

I attended my grandfather's church, the First Baptist Church of Amherstburg in Ontario, Canada. Escaped slaves originally built the church as a log cabin in the mid 1800s. It was one of the final stations of the Underground Railroad—the system whereby slaves traveled from safe house to safe house until they reached freedom in Canada. The North American Black Historical Museum around the corner from the church houses many of the artifacts from the church and tells the historical story of the slave trade and Underground Railroad. Pews that were replaced before I was born are in the museum along with the piano that I remember my mother playing hymns on during Sunday service. The museum also has three tombstones that were accidentally plowed up in what farmers believed to be an empty field. As it turned out, it used to be an old cemetery. One of those tombstones is that of my great-great grandfather, Robert Bayliss. While we have no proof, we like to think that he escaped through the Underground Railroad through the Amherstburg church. How amazing it would be if the descendent of former slave Robert Baylis married the Amherstburg preacher's daughter long after his death and journey to freedom.

Our church was so family oriented that each of the women at one time or another had a hand in raising us. Some were nurturing and made sure we were eating healthy; some told us when we weren't acting very ladylike; and most of them treated me like their own daughter since I played with their children. One particular church lady got everyone straight with her cane. She grew tomatoes and lived next door to the church. She often gave us some of her produce until it became unlawful to take vegetables and fruits across the border. Although she never had children of her own, she mothered, and disciplined, all of the children of the church. My girlfriend now laughs, "She yelled at us as if we were her own, and now she yells at my kids." I suppose I now appreciate her sternness.

As children we always sat with my grandmother while my mother, as the small church's musician, played the piano. My dad sat on the first pew next to her and the piano. Who knows, perhaps that's where he sat when they were dating.

My grandfather preached and was therefore in the pulpit and Lillian Granny took care of all four of her grandchildren. I was the oldest and then there was my cousin Terri who was almost four years younger than me. Her brother was three months older than my brother and they were both seven years younger than me. Lillian Granny always kept candy in her purse and we thought it was to keep us kids occupied in church. But watching her now in her eighties, I realize that she likes candy herself. Granny and Granddaddy were the quintessential grandparents from a time and place in Kentucky when men worked and women took care of the family and home. That was plenty of work for Granny and she did it well; she busied herself as a pastor's wife, working on several committees, and was a member of her neighborhood block club. She has remained an avid gardener well into her eighties in not only her yard, but also in those of her daughters and grandchildren.

As children, when we made too much noise during church, Lillian Granny had a three-step process to get us to behave. Along with the candy in her purse, she carried a narrow women's belt folded to purse size with a rubber band holding it together at the end. The first time we made noise, warning #1, she put the purse on her lap. The second time, warning #2, she took the belt out, placed it on her lap and gave us a stern look. If there was a third time, she had reflexes that would shave the hair off of mosquito knuckles. She'd grab the belt off of her lap and catch you on the leg and put it back into her purse, all in one fell swoop. The sting of the smack would make you want to yell, but you didn't dare—not in church.

I remember once when I was in middle school, we were playing and I knew that Terri and the boys were getting too loud, but never did I expect what was about to happen. Before

Granny could begin her warning system, my grandfather stopped his sermon and looked over in our pew and said, "Children. Please." I have never yet been more embarrassed in my life. After we quieted down, I moved to the pew in front to be away from them. After church Granddaddy wasn't mad, but I was embarrassed.

My grandfather baptized me when I was 14 years old. I remember what began as a warm spot in my heart became a burning desire to know the Lord better. Even at 14, as I listened to my grandfather's sermons about God's love and saving grace, I wanted to know and be a part of this blessed assurance of salvation. If I could be assured to have a friend to talk to about anything, a protector to keep me safe whether I was with my parents or not, and a comforter when life hurts, I wanted to sign up.

One Sunday morning I walked to the front of the church during the invitation to discipleship. I remember feeling my grandmother look at me. She used to always tell us that there is no walking during church service unless there is an emergency. And there were no emergencies during prayer, scripture reading, the sermon, offering or the invitation to join the church. So when I walked to the front I could imagine the stream of questions in her mind. She probably thought, "I know she's not walking during the invitation, so she must be joining the church." In front of the pulpit was my grandfather who gave me the right hand of fellowship and then a big hug.

On baptism Sunday, as was always done, Trustee Harris prepared the baptismal pool by running water through a hose into a tin pool accessed by lifting the pulpit floor. The baptism pool was constructed in the 1960s as an addition to the church that was built by slaves in the 1800s. If the aluminum siding (also an addition) was pulled away, as it is in the neighboring Amherstburg North American Black Historical Museum, you'd see the hand sewn log structure. Trustee Harris always filled the pool a few days in advance so that the water would warm at least to room temperature. In earlier years the pool was filled with river water, and before the pool was built, people were baptized in the Detroit River which separates the U.S. and Canada.

My mother played the piano of course, and I knew it was time when she played, "Take Me to the Water." My aunt, my mother's sister, went to the bathroom with me to help me get dressed in all white. My grandmother was busy helping my grandfather into his hip boots and robe. I met my grandfather at the entrance to the sanctuary and he looked at me this time as a grandfather and asked, "Are you ready?" I looked up at him proudly and said, "Yes, I am". He entered the pool first as my grandmother draped a white towel over his shoulder. Everyone gathered by the pool and began singing to my mother's soft piano playing, "Take me to the water, to be baptized."

We prayed as a normal part of the service, and he once again asked me if I was ready to accept the Lord as my personal savior. I answered yes and he proclaimed, "Having confessed the faith, I baptize you, my sister, in the name of the Father, the Son and Holy Ghost." He pinched my nose with his left hand and supported my body with his right arm. He lowered me into the watery grave and lifted me up anew.

Granddaddy wiped my face with the white towel that Lillian Granny draped across his shoulder. I recall the first face I saw after being baptized was that of my aunt. She was smiling with tears in her eyes. She covered me in a blanket and escorted me back to the bathroom to change. I remember being so excited and feeling so refreshed. Not just because the water was so cold, but I actually felt at that moment that my sins had been washed away. They would go out with the water when Trustee Harris siphoned out the water, back through the hose using gravity to empty the pool.

I told my aunt how I felt and she stopped with all of the blankets and towels and gave me a big hug. I'll never forget that moment. I'll never forget how she listened so intently to me.

The First Baptist Church of Amherstburg is a small church with about 20 members. Most of who belonged to one of 3-4 families. Because our church was so small, we each performed many functions at church. The ladies of the church held the Annual Calendar Tea. Each woman selected from a hat a month out of the year to decorate her table to reflect. January was decorated for New Year's Day, February for Valentine's Day, March for St. Patrick day, April for spring, May for Mother's Day, June celebrated weddings, July for summer or barbeques, August for Emancipation or when African-Canadian heritage was celebrated, September for fall and back to school, October when the Canadian Harvest Home (similar to the American Thanksgiving) is celebrated, November was winter, and of course December was Christmas. Each table was decorated with fine china and fabulous tea sandwiches and desserts. As I got older, my girlfriend and I became chairpersons for the Calendar Tea. Since I was in school and knew how to take notes, I became the church historian and took notes at the church meetings. For such a historic church, I felt extremely under-qualified, but I did the best I could.

Later when I was in college the commute to Amherstburg

was two hours from Ann Arbor. After a Saturday night of partying, Sunday's commute was like a cross-country road trip. I'd often make it in late so instead of sitting up front with my grandmother, I'd hold my head in my hands in the back pew. It's only now that I know that I wasn't fooling anyone.

High School Friendships

I had lots of friends in high school, but my two best friends in high school were Lisa and Marilyn. Lisa's father bought five acres in the country first and told my dad about it. So after growing up across the street from one another, we moved next door to one another. Our old school was predominantly black, and when we moved into the country, our school was 12% black. During our first year, February came and there was no mention of Black History Week (back then it was a week long). We had never heard of such a thing, and couldn't imagine that there'd be no mention of something which received national recognition! So we approached the administrators about the issue. They finally explained that if we wanted to make it an after-school activity, we could get a teacher as a sponsor. When we told our parents what the administrators said, they were appalled. My mother recalls talking to the principal from her job. She explained that the purpose of the national recognition was to teach all Americans about the contributions of African-Americans. She added that while many black students likely receive much of that education at home, the white students likely did not. She continued that to treat Black History Week like an after school activity doesn't allow the entire student body to participate and learn. Furthermore if this task is left up to two middle school girls, the other students won't learn enough. The administrators relented and we planned our

Black History Week program. Lisa and I were proud of our evening event in the media center for Black History Week; complete with the unveiling of a portrait drawn by my friend Lisa which she donated to the school.

I could always depend on Lisa through thick and thin. Once when the cheerleaders were selling candy in order to raise money for new cheerleading uniforms, I was my own best customer. Carrying chocolate bars with almonds, with crackles, and my personal favorite, with caramel filling, was too much for this diabetic to handle. I don't recall how many I ate, but in the middle of class my high blood sugar symptoms became worse than I ever recall. Besides cotton mouth, a headache and difficulty staying focused, I was nauseous. When I finally threw up, I asked to be excused from the rest of class. I had driven my mother to work and then drove myself to school. I knew I couldn't drive myself to the hospital, so I went to the office to find out which class Lisa was in. We both got permission to leave the school and Lisa drove me in my mother's car to the hospital.

Indeed my blood sugar was very high and I was dehydrated from throwing up. They gave me some insulin to lower my blood sugar and an IV to replace my fluids. The doctor explained that I was at the beginning stages of Diabetic Keytoacidosis (DKA).

We called my mother to tell her what had happened and that we had her car in Ann Arbor. She got a ride home and waited, probably not so patiently, for us to arrive home. When we arrived home, and Mom heard the whole story and she was sure I would be ok, she forbade me to ever sell candy again. Mom explained it as a temptation that I didn't need to have.

My other friend Marilyn did everything well. She did

alright academically, was an incredible athlete, was pretty, and of course all the guys liked her. She was a gymnast, a cheerleader, basketball player, diver, hurdler and she could have done more but there are only 24 hours in a day. She was amazing. She tried diving just to see if she could, and she was the best. I even managed to get an article published in the local newspaper that I wrote about Marilyn's abilities and ambition. We were good friends and didn't compete with one another because we had sort of an understanding: she was the athlete and I was the scholar. I was a member of the National Honor Society, a cheerleader, and played "at" softball. She played most sports at a varsity level and was an honor roll student. I was a better student and she was a better athlete.

I played softball my junior year in high school and made the JV team. Marilyn's sister, who was equally pretty and athletic, and her friend played varsity. One day after practice we stood around talking about how hot it was and how thirsty we were. Just then two guys from our high school showed up with a large thermos and paper cups. Midge (Marilyn's sister) asked if that was water. When they said sure, have some, we all got a cup of water. Before I got a chance to drink, the boys laughed and said that they urinated in the water. Midge spit out the water and began to chase one of the boys named Richard. They claimed that they were just kidding, that there wasn't urine in the water, but we never really knew. Little did I know then what a critical role Richard and urine would later play in my life.

We were leaders in high school. On graduation day my friends and I were decorated with honor cords and tassels as class officers, members of the student council and National Honor Society. Marilyn had lots of athletic awards and was even nominated as Home Coming Queen. We graduated in 1980 and registered to vote in school so that we could vote the following fall in our first Presidential election: The 1980 election of Ronald Reagan versus Jimmy Carter.

During my senior year of high school my grandfather, who was also my minister and spiritual leader, was diagnosed with lung cancer. He decided to proceed with surgery and so they removed his right lung. He recuperated with my grandmother at his side and even made my high school graduation. I was so thankful for God sparing him. I wanted to make him so proud when I attended the University of Michigan the following fall.

College Life

Hail to the Victors! After my senior year of high school I headed to the University of Michigan. Boy was I lucky as I look back on it. I applied to one school and got into one school. I don't know what would have happened if I didn't get in. Likewise I don't know what would have happened if I applied to other schools. I was recruited by Boston College, but my dad said that $9000 per term for out-of-state tuition was too much. It didn't matter to me, all my parents wanted was for me to get a good education, and I knew how proud my dad was of my cousins, his niece and nephew who also went to Michigan before me. I'll always remember attending my first U of M football game with my dad when I was a little girl. I of course had season tickets my freshman year and couldn't wait to take my dad. Every football Saturday, my roommate, Thea, and I invited someone, my dad, her nephew and my brother who were the same age, our mothers—we made it an event.

During the cold winter games of November, when we

went without family, we just took a stiff drink and huddled up to keep warm. I like to think of it as receiving a well rounded college education; complete with all that college and campus life had to offer.

I think it is impossible for college roommates not to become good friends, but Thea and I were like "peas and carrots". We even traveled to one another's house on the weekends to visit. I'll never forget the first time I spent the weekend at Thea's house. I was 18 years old and grown, so I thought, and my parents traveled over an hour to meet Thea's mother before I spent the night. Our parents became good friends too.

Over the years, we shared expenses, saved one another from the wrong guy and my roommate even agreed to accompany me on a date when I didn't want to go out with the guy alone. And no one at that point in my life, since my mom, had sacrificed so much for my health. At 2 a.m. after complaining all evening of a backache, we walked down the street to the U of M Hospital. The Emergency Room doctors said I had a kidney infection. I should drink lots of water and take the antibiotics as prescribed. Thea waited for me in uncomfortable plastic chairs in the waiting room. She said next time she'd just bring a book or something and get studying done rather than try to sleep in those orange plastic chairs.

Thea did right by planning for the next time because indeed there was a next time. Thea and I went to her friend's party in her home town. Boy did we have fun. I danced so hard that I thought I pulled a muscle. In the car I continued to be in pain, and so she agreed that we should go to the nearest ER. Sure enough the doctors said it was a kidney infection again, and gave me my usual antibiotic. Thea and I played hard, but we worked hard academically as well.

With all the hard work and erratic schedule, my doctors felt that I needed a blood sugar control tune up and hospitalized me for a week to regulate my blood sugar. In the meantime, grades were mailed home. My dad visited the hospital with my grades in hand. I got As, Bs, and Cs, but I also got a D in statistics. I hoped for compassion from my professor. I took refuge under my hospital sheets as my father read them to me. My dad knew better; I wasn't at all sick. My dad said, "I don't pay for Ds. So you better figure it out and make a change."

I always brought guys home to meet my folks. Not so much as a formal event, but my parents just always ended up meeting them. They never offered judgment, at least not to me. Not until I brought home Gary. Gary followed me home to drop off my car because I ended up getting too many parking tickets with it on campus. My dog, Daisy, who was a sheep dog growled at Gary and jumped up on him. Although this was the second time my dad met Gary, he said to me later, "We're seeing an awful lot of Gary these days." Dad didn't want his daughter to get too involved before completing her education.

The way Gary and I met was the most creative way any man has approached me. I had never been pursued with such thoughtfulness and planning. Gary and I were in the same calculus class. When the professor handed back the first test he had to call our names because he didn't know any of us. And so Gary knew my name. At that time, you could call the university Student Locator with just a name and get a phone number. And so Gary used the Student Locator to call me. He said he missed class and wanted to borrow my notes. He came to my dorm room and copied my notes. He didn't look any different than all the other white boys in that big lecture hall, so I never knew whether he missed class or not. Weeks later, Gary did it again; he copied my notes. After class one Friday, he asked if I'd like to have dinner with him.

I was surprised and told him that I was going home for the weekend and couldn't. Gary was persistent and asked another Friday. Finally I relented. He took me to dinner at Weber's, a restaurant I hadn't been to since my parents paid (I mean took me).

About a week later, as I walked toward my dorm room after class, the white girls across the hall were holding some Valentine's Day flowers and said a very handsome man left them for me. They teased me over and over again about how handsome he was. That was really code for he was white and why on earth did he give them to me and not them. I opened the card and they were from Gary for Valentine's Day. He called later and asked if I received the pink and white roses. I told him yes. He asked how many were there. I told him it looks to be a dozen and a half. He said, "Oh no, there should be only 17". As I counted, there were only 17 and I told him. He said, "Do you know what the number 17 represents?" I said no. He explained that he had known me for 17 days and that's why he sent 17 roses. Needless to say, I was impressed. So Thea and I let him hang out.

If going from a predominantly black elementary school to a predominantly white middle and high school was a change, the University of Michigan was less diverse than high school. At Michigan, black students always spoke to one another in passing, whether they knew one another or not. It was a recognition that said, because there are so few of us, we must respect and recognize one another. It made us all a kindred spirit. There was even a talent show at one of the north campus dormitories that showcased the talents other than academic skill that Michigan's black students possessed. The event was a tough show to get into because there were so many talented people. One of my roommates, who later became a Harvard trained physician, played piano as another woman sang. One student who hosted the show as a comedian later became an attorney and most recently a Hollywood writer and director. His talent was so evident even then.

Thea and I finished undergrad and I continued work on my master's degree at Michigan in Public Policy and Thea went to Penn State University to graduate with a master's degree in Speech and Language Pathology. I had new roommates. One was a year younger than me and the other, on track to graduate with me, was applying to medical schools. She was accepted to all three and attended Harvard. She practiced interview questions and sincerely asked us what we thought would be her weakness as a physician. I recall receiving a phone call for her at 7 a.m. All three of us were up and preparing for class, but we weren't used to the phone ringing that early. It was for my roommate preparing for medical school and we heard her official voice answering questions about why she wanted to study medicine. I remember one of her most distressing questions wasn't about medicine or her abilities at all. It was, if she was such a good musician (she played piano) and writer (she won writing awards), why then did she want to practice medicine?

Besides her obvious academic talent, she composed music and was a devout Seventh Day Adventist. She wrote and performed a song for a friend's wedding. I admired her discipline in all areas of her life. She was an excellent student and never studied beyond sundown on Friday. She read her Bible and ate no pork. Wanting to emulate her discipline, I became vegetarian—for a few years.

One day I came home from class in the middle of the afternoon and my roommate relayed the message that my mother called and our house was on fire. In shock and not quite knowing what to do, I called home. The line was busy—of course, it was on fire. I asked if there was more and she didn't know anything more. I called the neighbor's house; Lisa's mom answered and said my mom was there. Mom assured me that everyone was ok, but the house was about gone. I grabbed my keys and walked a few blocks to my car and drove home. It normally took about 30 minutes to drive home, but that day I think I made it in about 15 minutes. As I drove home, I recalled that my mother, father and brother were ok, but I didn't ask about our dog, Daisy. Sure enough, my mom was crying frantically at Lisa's house and our dog, Daisy lay on the floor, just fine. It probably seemed strange that I was so happy to see the dog and just said hi to my mom; but I knew that my family was ok—it was Daisy that I wasn't sure about.

Our pet bird was, as my brother described, "Parakeet under glass". After the fire the only thing left of our piano was the music wire. My parents stayed at Lillian Granny and Granddaddy's house that night after stopping at a convenience store to get toiletries and another store to buy clothes for the next day. We spent the next few days trying to salvage what we could from the fire. All of my high school memories, varsity letters, yearbooks and pictures were gone.

Whenever I went home on the weekend, I always borrowed

a sweater, shirt or sox from my mom, dad or brother. I even borrowed the mutton coat that my dad bought my mom before they got married to wear to a ball. So after the fire, I was able to pack up a full suit case of their belongings that I had at my apartment. They were surprised to know I had borrowed so much and not returned it.

A Well-Rounded Education

Thea and I met some friends in the graduate school of public policy who ate at our dorm. I was studying political science and was interested in their studies. We invited them to go to a party with us across campus. As graduate school students, they lived off campus and drove to our dorm to meet us. Being the "hostesses with the mostest," we offered them a drink before we left. In the back of our clothes closet was our alcohol storage. One drink led to another and another and before we knew it we were watching one of the guys climb light poles on our way to the party and I somehow forgot to change shoes before leaving for the party and managed to wear Thea's house slippers. We walked to and from the party and made it there safely and back—house slippers and all.

Once we were celebrating the end of the term—not as if we needed a reason to celebrate, but this time we had one. Thea and I weren't roommates, but still hung out together. Thea and I went to the bar with a guy who wanted to take me out, and as a precaution, I said both of us or none of us. He took us to his favorite spot and ordered us Harvey Wall Bangers. We enjoyed them but didn't know that he ordered us double shots of alcohol in the drinks. Further, we hadn't eaten dinner yet. I got sick to the stomach before dinner came and being rehearsed in hospital runs, Thea knew just what to do. He paid the bill and threw me over his shoulder and then into his daddy's yellow Cadillac where I threw up all over the white interior. We went to my apartment and then Thea said as if she were Batman, "To the Emergency room."

Being responsible, my new roommates called my parents to meet us at the emergency room. Of course, mine and Thea's plan was to get in and out without my parents knowing we were drunk. I remember the cute intern saying that my blood sugar was fine, however my blood alcohol level was 3.0, but he didn't think he had to pump my stomach. Meanwhile, Thea was busted fumbling with her broken glasses and trying not to breathe alcohol on my parents (as if they didn't know that we had been drinking).

The next morning I remember waking up in my grandmother's bedroom at my parents' house (my father's mother lived with us but was visiting her daughters for the weekend). I was on top of the covers and fully dressed. I wondered how I got there and didn't remember driving home. I went upstairs to my parents' room, sat at the end of the bed and asked them, "What happened?" My mother looked down in embarrassment and my Dad said, "You were drunk, and we brought you home. It's a good thing your roommates called. And that Thea nearly got me drunk from giving me a hug when we got there. I just have one thing to say: I've been drunk before, and in all my days, I've always come home with two shoes!" It seems in the scuffle and throwing me over his shoulder, I lost a shoe.

After a much-needed sleep I borrowed shoes from my mom and went back to school. Early the next spring, after the snow melted, I found my other rust-colored suede shoe in the apartment parking lot.

I often look back on those times and reflect that it's amazing that we're still alive. I also think, even after all that has happened since, I wouldn't change a single thing.

Diabetes – A Family Affair

My mother started having symptoms of constant thirst and frequent urination. She decided that since she was under the stress of having just lost her father and losing our home in a fire, this could very possibly be adult onset (Type II) diabetes. She went to the doctor and explained that by raising a child with diabetes for then about 13 years; she not only understood the risk factors but the symptoms of diabetes too. Indeed, when the doctor checked her blood, she, too, was diabetic. Because my mother felt that it was her diagnosis, she asked that he only charge the insurance company half price for the visit.

At first she wasn't insulin dependent, and then she started taking insulin. No doubt her pancreas took its last insulin producing breath. Now we were both insulin dependent. While she was in the hospital being regulated, I went to work in Lansing as part of my graduate studies internship. I came home to the apartment my family was staying in for the balance of my brother's school year. While my mother was in the hospital, I planned to help my dad and brother get ready for the week and cook them a meal. When I entered the apartment, it looked like a war zone. Clothes were all over the living room and there was not even one clean dish in the kitchen. So I ran the dishwasher, took the dirty clothes to the laundry room and washed them. I cleaned and disinfected the apartment and ironed enough shirts for dad to wear to work for the next week. For dinner that night they decided that it was best that they finish up the hard salami, onions and

Limburger cheese they had the day before. The Limburger cheese explained why the apartment smelled like sweat sox. I concluded that they were pretending to be bachelor room-mates while Mom was away. Feeling confident that they could make it another week, and that my mother wouldn't come home from the hospital to a total disaster, I left to finish my summer internship in Lansing, MI.

❀ ❀ ❀

Chapter Two

To Have and to Hold
From This Day Forward

When I first told my dad that my boyfriend Steve and I were thinking of getting married, he said, "Oh, well I better look at him in a different light!" Dad was so used to meeting every guy that I dated, that he never knew if it was someone special or not. He continued joking by comparing him to other guys I dated. According to Daddy, the beer distributor always had samples of exotic beers for him to try; the guy who worked for the Detroit Tigers could get him good tickets. But Steve is a funeral director and according to Daddy, "What's Steve gonna get me? A good funeral?"

Although our engagement wasn't official with a ring, my mother and I shopped reception halls. Once we decided on one, we made an appointment for my dad (with the check book) and Steve to join us. We had to make a deposit to hold the date. It made sense to meet at my dad's office, and so we did. Before we left, my dad asked Steve into his office and closed the door. My mom and I couldn't hear what was going on, but we heard lots of fist slamming and bangs on the door. My dad opened the door and said, "OK, we're ready to go."

At that point, we set a date, but Steve hadn't given me an engagement ring yet. He said he showed my dad the receipt, but other than that, I still, 20 years later, don't know what he said.

Retinopathy

Two months before our wedding, Steve and I were at a friend's house when I noticed that I saw a red spot in my right eye, regardless of what I looked at. The next day I scheduled an appointment with my ophthalmologist who referred me to a retinal specialist. He explained that I had proliferative retinopathy.

Proliferative retinopathy is when blood vessels become weakened in the retina of the eye and leak blood into the vitreous fluid. Retinopathy is a complication of diabetes. The body's natural defense is to grow new blood vessels to replace the leaking ones. However, the new blood vessels are weaker than the ones they replace and soon leak themselves. Retinal Specialists use laser to destroy the weaker blood vessels and reroute blood through the stronger ones instead. Because my blood vessels leaked, the blood in my vitreous (the jelly like substance in the middle of the eye ball) formed a blood clot. The clot affected my vision by creating a shadow blocking out 50% of my vision in my right eye.

My retinal specialist explained that there are two treatments for this condition. One is to do nothing and the body heals itself by reabsorbing the blood out of the vitreous fluid. The second involves surgery by removing the vitreous fluid from the eye and replacing it with synthetic fluid. He recommended the surgery because waiting for the clot to reabsorb would cause scar tissue to pull the retina away from the back of the eye, causing at best, distortion in my vision. To help me decide, he asked me to see other doctors in his practice. One of his partners recommended surgery and the other recommended doing nothing. I chose the solution that would allow me to live the most normal life. I chose surgery.

I was scared. Although retinopathy wasn't at the top of my list of long-term complications of diabetes that I hoped never to get, I was still scared. The blood clot appeared as a shadow or dark cloud in my field of vision. I couldn't drive because glare at night bothered me and with one eye closed, I hadn't yet learned to compensate.

The surgery was done under a microscope but didn't take long. The midnight nurse came to help me to the bathroom and to change my bandages. When she got them off, I was surprised that I could see completely. I guess I thought I wouldn't be able to see for some time after the surgery. I was discharged from the hospital the next day. My fiancé, Steve, was a funeral director, and so it was commonplace if convenient for him to complete errands in the hearse. My discharge time was 11 a.m. Eleven in the morning is prime time for funerals, and this day was no different. As soon as the funeral service was complete, he swung by the hospital to take me home in the hearse! The nurse who wheeled me out to the pick-up area didn't move until she saw my fiancée get out of the hearse. She said, "Oh, that's your ride," as she chuckled and others looked on with a puzzled stare.

After some daily eye drops and soreness, everything was back to normal. Almost normal—documented in our wedding album is the fact that I had no eyelashes on my right eye. The doctor said not to use eye drops for redness; however, he prescribed something that would take out the redness to be used for the wedding day only. And so, the later the night got, the more bloodshot my right eye became in the pictures.

Diabetes and Marriage

In 1989 I married the man who has been here by my side in sickness and in health. Our wedding day was beautiful. We had seven bridesmaids and seven groomsmen, a junior bridesmaid, flower girl and ring bearers who walked with them as well. Steve's bachelor party was the night before the wedding at our friend's house that lived across the street from my house. My cousin, who was also in the wedding, and I pulled our hair into baseball caps and put on big sweat shirts and tried to get into the party. One of the attendants was so drunk that he almost let us in. The host recognized us and pushed us out of the door. We laughed all the way back across the street. As we began to cross the street, a car pulled up with girls dressed in furs and high-heeled shoes. We chose to ignore it.

Waiting back at my house was my dad. He went to the bachelor party for a while, but felt like he was cramping my brother's style—not Steve's or his friends', but his son's. Steve spent the night at my house and I went home with my Daddy.

The next morning Steve sent me a dozen red roses. My cousin arranged for a hair stylist to come to the house to do my hair around my veil. I ate at about 1 p.m. to have a flat stomach by 5 p.m., but especially so that I didn't have an insulin reaction in the middle of the ceremony. We joked that if I was sick, maybe I couldn't get the vows out.

When we arrived at the church by limousine, Dad and I waited in the basement for our turn. We watched through the basement window as latecomers arrived. We noted business acquaintances, family and friends. There were more than 500 people at our wedding and 350 at the reception. My dad looked me in the eye and said to me in his sincere tone, "You look real pretty." I hugged him and said, "Thanks, Dad." He said, "You know, we can still leave and you don't have to do this." I smiled and we both laughed.

We went to Hawaii for our honeymoon. The doctor said to be careful with the sun, so I went sunglasses shopping! My vision improved and I learned to compensate for the slight distortion, although my eye muscles were slightly weakened in that eye. I told my new husband that I put my retinal specialist right up there next to Jesus because Jesus also gave sight to the blind. We laughed.

Married life was great and Steve was glad to get regular homemade meals–meals he used to have to ask his adopted sister he worked with to include him in on. Her husband later told me he didn't know whether to claim Steve on his income tax or hope one day he found another place to eat.

My dog Max had his own introduction for Steve, the newcomer in the house. Max tried to tell Steve that, "I do sleep next to mommy in the bed." And when I made my first married meal of fried chicken leg and thigh quarters, green beans and corn, Max snatched Steve's plate off of the table and ate the chicken. Steve's favorite is chicken. Max had a look on his face as if to say, "... In case you thought you were the man of the house, let me show you." Max came to realize that Steve wasn't leaving, so they became friends. Steve was feeling outnumbered with Max and me. So he got an antisocial alley cat from his mother. Whenever guests came over, Missey the cat ran to hide. Many of our friends never knew that we had a cat.

Diabetes and Pregnancy

Our wedding ceremony began, "Jacqueline and Stephen, feeling incomplete alone . . ." Well this time the two of us felt not quite complete together, and on August 2nd, 1991 at 2:21 p.m. the Lord cured that incomplete feeling by blessing us with a son, Stevie.

I recall during a hospital stay in the '70s, the doctor's encouraging news that medical progress has now enabled diabetic women to have children. Since I was 7 when my endocrinologist told me this, it didn't seem important. However when I was ready, being Type 1 diabetic meant that my pregnancy was anything but a "normal" pregnancy, if there is such a thing. My pregnancy required close attention from the start. In the beginning, the challenge was to keep my body healthy; kind of like an incubator for little Stephen. It was then, at 11weeks gestation that the doctors prepared us for the rough road ahead—the risks on my life and the baby's life were high. The work would be hard, but if we could keep our faith in God strong, the reward would be wonderful, my perinatoligist explained.

My doctor was a robust and jovial man with an amazing reputation for positive outcomes in high-risk pregnancies. I recall being told that he himself was a premature twin. Both he and his twin were doctors. I recall him telling me and Steve when I was hospitalized at 11 weeks gestation, that if we did all that he asked that he would do all he could medically to produce a positive outcome. That turned out to include canceling airline tickets and a hotel stay that my girlfriend and

I bought to surprise our husbands for their birthdays. The doctor said that it was too early in my pregnancy to fly.

The level of health monitoring reminded me of my days when I was first diagnosed diabetic. With each new trimester of my pregnancy the challenges grew tougher. My insulin requirements, moods and health changed as the baby grew. Soon I felt like I had a specialist for every organ in my body—a perinatologist for my unborn child and my pregnancy, a retinal specialist for my eyes, a nephrologists for my kidneys, a gastrointestinal surgeon for my liver, a hematologist for my blood disorders, a neurologist for the nerve pain in my back, a cardiologist for my pregnancy induced hypertension and an internist to monitor my diabetes. I also had teaching nurses and dieticians.

With each new challenge my prayers became longer and more frequent. They always began, "Dear Lord, thank you for the many blessings that you've bestowed upon me thus far—I have so much to be thankful for". And then I'd ask Him to heal my body and protect my unborn child.

Alas, the final stretch of the pregnancy began on July 8, 1991 when I entered the hospital for the fourth and final time of the pregnancy. At 5'4", I weighed 180 pounds, was very swollen and my blood pressure was 150/100. My doctor was very concerned that I might be developing toxemia and he ordered complete bed rest while in the hospital. During the first two weeks I lost nine pounds of water weight and began feeling better. However, the doctor felt it best for me to remain hospitalized for the duration of the pregnancy. This final stretch would be a delicate tightrope walk balancing my life and that of my unborn child. Monitoring my health meant each day the lab would draw blood work and do a urinalysis which tested my kidney function, liver enzymes, creatinine clearance and blood clotting ability. Monitoring the baby's health meant daily fetal heart monitoring (a procedure where they hooked a machine up to my belly to monitor the baby's heart rate), daily kick counts to make sure the baby was moving, and 3 ultra sounds and biophysical profiles per week. During the biophysical profiles they scored the baby's performance with 2 points each for size or circumference of the head, leg movement, arm movement, and diaphragm movement—meaning the baby was taking practice breaths. At this point the baby's heart rate was good, movement was excellent and he scored 8 out of 8 on each biophysical profile. However, the pole wasn't balanced on my end of the stick. I had increased protein spillage in my urine, and high levels of creatinine—both indications of kidney disease. Also my liver enzymes were elevated and the doctors worried about hepatitis. Anemic as well, I began to feel tired. The aches and pains began to take its toll. A sharp pain in my lower back that resonated around my left side brought me to tears. My prayers were to be faithful and that God knows how much I can bear.

The doctor felt that I should be more closely monitored since my stress could send me into premature labor, therefore he moved me to the High Risk Labor & Delivery room. After ruling out a kidney infection, the neurologist concluded that it was probably a pinched nerve caused by the baby. We could not verify it because an x-ray would be a risk to the baby. He ordered a night of codeine and physical therapy to relax me.

I had the same roommate in the hospital for 2 ½ weeks. She too was one of my doctor's regular patients. Her reason for hospitalization was dangerous hypertension, and she had miscarried twice. One of the miscarriages ended when she went into pre-term labor and had seizures because her blood pressure shot up so high. The baby was born at about 2 pounds, however, later the baby died. Therefore, this hospitalization was stressful for her as well. When the time came for her to have her baby I could empathize with her anxiety. We had talked about our faith and the Lord, so when they came to wheel her down to labor and delivery at 5 a.m. for her scheduled induced labor, I told her I would be here praying for her, and I did. I asked God to wrap His arms around her and to bring her and the baby safely through the delivery.

Even when the going gets tough, there is always someone else in need of prayer. I prayed hard for my hospital roommate, her baby, and her husband. After unproductive labor, she had an emergency cesarean section and the Lord brought mother, baby and husband through just fine.

My testing continued and the doctor grew more concerned about my health. But he did not want to deliver the baby if his lungs weren't mature enough to breathe on his own. A baby's lungs are the last to develop. The doctor scheduled me for an amniocentesis that would better determine if the baby was mature. It was his judgment that as soon as the baby was mature, he should deliver it to preserve my health. At the same time I think he scheduled the surgery for two days after the test—assuming the baby was mature.

Finally at 36 weeks, the doctor decided it was time for the C-section. I called my Mom first because she was farthest away and because she is MOM. I called my husband second because he had just left the hospital. I called my Dad last because he was closest and he was excited. My Dad arrived first and I told him that my husband hadn't arrived yet and so he'll have to go into the delivery room with me. He said "no,

no, no, my job is to get coffee for the doctor. Where's Steve?"
And he started to walk out looking for him. I told him I was
joking so that he would calm down.

When we went into the operating room I was strapped to
the table with a blood pressure cuff on one arm and an IV in
the other. I received the saddle block and the resident began
to make some cuts. He nervously asked if I felt anything. His
question made me more nervous about him than the delivery
itself. I thought to myself, "If it hurt, you'd certainly know
it." The doctor in the operating room had the radio playing
Temptations oldies. It was great to finally have some fun with
a medical procedure.

The doctors saw in the ultra sound that my son was
breached and decided on how to lift him out of my stomach.
I later found child birth was easier to explain to my son when
I described his own birth via C-section. Somehow it seemed
easier to tell than that of natural childbirth—especially to a
young boy. I was afraid that they wouldn't get my husband in
the operating room in time. Just then he walked in through
the door. I had seen other expectant fathers dressed in their
green hospital scrubs. But Steve couldn't be just like all the
rest. He had washed and pressed his old white hospital jacket
with his name and Cardiology (from his previous research job)
on the lapel. He wore that buttoned up as if it were 30 degrees
in the hospital, on top of his scrubs.

Of course with a month to prepare for this glorious
moment, I had the camera already in my hospital room. I
told my husband to take pictures with it like the ones I'd seen
from other mothers in my doctor's office. So I asked him,
"Are you ready? Do you have the camera?" And he nervously
said, "No". Since my son would be born only once, I decided

that now wasn't the time to argue, and let it pass. The room was filled with nine medical professionals. There was a set of doctors, nurses and anesthesiologists for me and another for my son. After I thought about it, it certainly made sense. If something went wrong, we each had a team available to work on us individually, so no doctor had to decide which patient to treat. The room was full and there were certainly no secrets— meaning my hospital gown was open to all in the room.

Finally the doctor pulled Stephen out back first, with his head facing down. The doctors rushed him onto a table and cleared his mouth. I heard him cry and knew that everything was ok. It's amazing how the whole room waits to hear that cry, and once it is belted out, everyone sighs. After cleaning him up, they put him into an incubator and wheeled him out of the operating room. The doctor explained that they would take him to the neonatal intensive care unit and perform further tests.

Before my husband went into the operating room, my father instructed Steve that his first order of business after the baby was born was to step into the hall and signal one finger for a girl and two fingers for a boy. Steve had forgotten and besides it wouldn't have been practical. I got my first good glance at my baby when he was wheeled out in the incubator. He looked so big for a newborn. The doctor said he weighed 6 pounds and 11 ounces, and 19.5 inches long. The doctor was surprised that he was such a healthy weight born at 36 weeks gestation. Since I had a month to wait in the hospital before Stephen was born, I had calculated in pounds the parameters based on the ultra sounds—yeah, talk about your boredom. I asked my father for the conversion factor for kilograms to pounds, so I knew according to the ultra sound weight estimates that the lowest he would weigh was five pounds, ten ounces and the highest was about seven pounds, two ounces. I was happy that my calculations were accurate.

I tried to have a tender moment with my husband, as the excitement seemed to wind down. I looked over and Steve was a peculiar shade of lime green. I couldn't believe this man who observed several open heart surgeries, watched his friend's open heart surgery and who now is a funeral director and sews back autopsy cases, was turning green at the sight of our son being born. He explained that he'd never seen his wife opened up that way, that's why it was so shocking.

As the doctors sewed me up, I began to feel nauseous myself. The anesthesiologist reached for a pan and said for me to lean left and throw up just below my armpit. So I let her rip. When I arrived to the recovery room I was freezing and starting to feel some of the pain from surgery. The nurse covered me with lots of warm blankets from the warmer and gave me something for the pain. By this time, lots of people made it to the hospital. My mom made it from work before I went into the operating room and couldn't believe she was a grandmother. My girlfriend was there with her children. Another girlfriend and her daughter and her daughter's boyfriend came to the hospital.

What a joyous time it was. All of my hard work and preparation had come to a crescendo—my son was born.

At birth Stephen's blood sugar was 40. Normal is 70 to 120. The doctor explained that he was so used to high blood sugars when he was in my diabetic body that his little pancreas was continuing to work overtime. He said we'll feed him decreasing amounts of glucose until his blood sugar normalizes. Sure enough his blood sugar normalized. Because he was a premature baby and the lungs are the last to develop, he was on 100% oxygen in a tent. After a few days he was on no oxygen at all.

The doctors left me in labor and delivery to recuperate and reduce pain medicine while getting my blood sugars back under control after so much change to my body. For most surgeries and for this one, I was taken off of long acting insulin and given only short acting regular insulin several times during the day. The next day, my doctor left orders for the resident to calculate what my new requirements should be and to start the long acting. When I took my insulin I noticed the dose was only short acting and asked the nurse why I wasn't taking any long acting insulin. She said that it wasn't written in the orders and so I took the dose prescribed. It seemed like not enough but perhaps they knew better than me. Indeed by afternoon, my blood sugar was high and near 400. I overheard the doctor scolding the resident for not giving me long acting insulin. We treated the high blood sugar with lots of shots of short acting insulin.

While I was regulating my blood sugars, it rarely dawned on me that I had a son that I should get ready to care for. In fact, the nurses asked if I wanted to go to the Neonatal Intensive Care unit and feed him. I asked if they had bottles and she said, "Yes", so I asked her to ask them to feed him, I couldn't move yet—I was tired and sore. I lay in the bed and thought what a lazy mother am I, and drifted off to sleep.

The next day when Steve came to the hospital, we went down to feed our son together. My mother took pictures. Little did I know (or care for that matter) that my hair stood up like Don King's. The only difference was that mine had light brown streaks instead of gray.

Later that night, I moved back to my regular room on the floor. My doctor came in to check on me. But this time, instead of standing at the end of my bed, he sat on the side. He still had on his Operating Room hat and shoes. He asked how I was doing. I thought it was odd that he would visit so late in the day. I told him I was fine. And while it was a check up call, it was more an opportunity for him to rest and reflect on positive matters. He explained that he had two women that he was trying not to deliver C-section and had done several earlier that day. Although we were different religions (my doctor was Jewish), he commented on how wonderful it was that Stephen wasn't on a ventilator. He fully expected when he delivered Stephen that he would need a ventilator. He said that, "If you weren't religious before, you have to believe that only God could do such a thing." It felt so comforting that my doctor was feeling thankful to God as well.

Juggling Diabetes, Motherhood and Working

The doctors were ready to release Stevie from neonatal intensive care and send him home. I still needed to stabilize my blood sugar and make sure all my organs were functioning the way they should. My roommate's new baby was discharged before she was and I was nervous that they might do the same to me. Her husband had two other children at home and a new baby wasn't new to him. The thought of my husband, an only child himself, home alone with my new baby would make me escape from the hospital by tying sheets together and scaling down the outside of the building. It was enough that he was caring for our cat and dog alone. I told the pediatrician after he examined Stevie to please hold off on discharging him until I was discharged. He said he would wait until Friday. That became my target – to convince my doctors that I was ready to be discharged on Friday. It all worked out and we both went home with the new dad on Friday. As I left the hospital, I was having an insulin reaction, so Stevie's first trip in the car included a stop at the drive thru at McDonalds.

I arrived home from the hospital a week after giving birth. It was nice to get home to a quiet house and get used to my new family. A nurse recommended that my husband bring a soiled diaper home a week before my son and I arrived for the cat and dog to smell and they wouldn't be curious when we brought home the baby. So when we walked through the door my dog Max and the cat Missey weren't interested in what was in the bundle of blankets at all. The nurse was right – they weren't curious at all.

When they say that mother instincts don't just click right in, I found out exactly what they meant. Up until then, I was going through the motions caring for my child. There was so much family and friends around me that I couldn't fail or fully appreciate this awesome responsibility. Finally one afternoon I looked at my baby in my arms and thought about what God had brought me through to have this wonderful life in my life. I also thought about what the doctors said about me having children when I was first diagnosed with diabetes. They told me how unlikely it was for me to carry a baby full term, if in fact I was able to get pregnant. I held my baby close to my heart and began to cry and pray.

The doctors said that I was spilling significant amounts of protein and prescribed a drug to prolong my kidney function (he said) for 7 years. I didn't think much of it, but took the pill faithfully along with some vitamins.

Weeks later an old friend of mine visited to see my new baby. He was awe struck at the thought of me being a mother. Steve came home from work just as my friend was getting ready to leave. I introduced them and as it turned out they were fraternity brothers. After my friend left, Steve asked if I used to date him. Surprised at his question, I told him well, kind of. We were more friends than anything and I attended his company functions with him. His bosses thought I was his girlfriend. That was a strange question for Steve to ask seemingly from nowhere. I asked him why he asked. He said that he noticed that my dog Max didn't bark at him but instead just lay at his feet. And my friend didn't appear to be bothered by it. I laughed and told Steve that if I were trying to do something wrong, I guess Max would tell it!

Breast-feeding worked for about two months. Fortunately I had a good nurse who explained that if it becomes too stressful for mom, then it is too stressful for the baby. Indeed it became too stressful. I worried that I wasn't producing enough milk—even though his weight proved he was thriving. Although I bought a pump, I could never seem to pump reserves. I arrived back at work when Stephen was three months old, and I still couldn't control leaks without looking like I had sweat socks in my bra. Taking the nurse's advice, I decided to end the frustration for us both and he went to bottle-feeding. Boy did I feel better. Feeding him every other hour was difficult on my body too. What I learned was that breast-feeding burns as much energy as riding a bicycle. No one explained to me, but constant insulin reactions taught me that I had to eat a snack before I started to breast-feed. The worst insulin reaction I've ever had in my life happened my first night home from the hospital with my new baby. My son woke up in the middle of the night to eat and Steve brought him to me in bed to breast feed. After feeding him I told Steve that my blood sugar felt low, so he went to the kitchen to get me something to eat. When he came back I had laid the baby down and was beginning to convulse. At that time I didn't have instant glucose in the house so he got the next best thing—grape juice concentrate from the freezer. He put a cup of warm water in a glass with the concentrate to melt the ice. I drank the syrup and felt better within minutes. It was then that I realized that in order to be the best mother I could, would mean that I had to be the healthiest mother I could. I began to take my diabetes control a lot more seriously.

While I was on maternity leave from Lewis Metal Stamping, Black Enterprise Magazine featured my father on the cover of their magazine. A local freelance reporter wrote the two-page article inside. I hated that I missed all of the excitement. I also missed making sure that everything was in order, including what my dad chose to wear. When I returned to work, there had been a few changes. We had a new receptionist who occasionally wore her sister's jacket that proclaimed her to be the "Da-Da Captain." For some reason I didn't think it stood for the Detroit Auto Dealers Association, nor did I want to know. After a few weeks, I could take it no longer. Her slang and unprofessional dress wasn't good for business. Meanwhile a friend of Steve's visited and mentioned that his wife was looking for a new job. We interviewed her and found that she had the right stuff and so she became our administrative assistant, and more.

A natural progression from quoting new business was to work in sales and marketing. So I went to customer seminars, met customers and planned for future business. My dad was so open with his work that whatever area I wanted to dabble in, he would let me. He let me explore almost whatever I wanted to. The company turned 10 years old and I planned an open house. We had golf shirts and hats for employees and customers and visitors. When it came time to meet the General Motor's Target for Excellence business requirement, I spear headed that effort. I met with GM personnel for months preparing for our two-day audit. I prepared (with my best U of M training) an elaborate presentation to make on the last day for the auditors. The guy from GM whom I'd been preparing for the audit with and had become friends with stopped me as I began pulling my transparencies out and said, "We've seen enough, I don't need a big presentation." I didn't argue because this audit was important for future business. We passed the audit with recommendations for future improvement. We were elated with our accomplishment. My customer friend knew I'd planned a big presentation for the end, and for years we laughed at how he wouldn't let me deliver it. He promised one day to finally listen to it—but he never did.

Early Elementary Parenting

After my son was in preschool for a year, and I learned to juggle the responsibilities of work and home, I moved my son into a Montessori elementary school. We attended the new student day before school started. As my husband and son visited inside the classroom, I went outside to look at the playground. Outside was a Korean mother who sat quietly on the swing set. We each introduced ourselves and it turned out we were both mothers of sons in the same classroom.

Several weeks after that I went shoe shopping for my son and noticed him playing with another child in the same school uniform. Just then, I noticed the same Korean mother walking toward me laughing. I shook her hand and she too said hello. She explained that she was laughing because her son Daniel kept telling her that he plays with his best friend

Stephen Kemp in school. As a preschooler, he didn't enunciate the "p" at the end of Kemp. So she asked Daniel if his friend was Korean and he answered yes. When the children began playing at the shoe store, Daniel said to her, "Mom, this is my friend Stephen Kim." I laughed too and we each continued shopping while they played.

For months to come, each time we reviewed the kids' work, each child described the other one as being his "best friend." While Daniel's mother and I thought that this was an extraordinary friendship, it was probably par for the course at the school because of its extraordinary diversity. Each classroom had an almost equal number of several nationalities or races. The school was comprised of seemingly equal numbers of black children, white children, Indian children, Asian children, Chaldean children, Jewish children and more. It was such a perfect world that it seemed to be by design. My son stayed there until he graduated from 5th grade.

It wasn't until one Easter Sunday morning when Stevie complained about wearing a suit and tie to church that I understood the true value of his diverse education. He told me that it wasn't fair that he had to wear a suit and tie, that his friend of Asian Indian descent didn't wear one to temple. As I searched for an explanation beyond that wearing new clothes symbolized the resurrected life of Jesus Christ, I realized that his friend's cultural diversity wasn't taught in school. While the school mentions cultural differences and notes Easter, Passover, Christmas, Chanukah, Ramadan and Kwanza, they don't typically discuss daily practices. I realized that what my son learned, he learned on the playground and not in the classroom. And only by filling a school with such diversity do you make way for cultural learning and sharing. What a benefit. He learned more than what could be taught in the classroom about how the world works, naturally, during play.

Diversity was an issue for his education that I thought was nice, but if a school didn't have it but was academically strong, perhaps it would be ok. I felt that way until I learned the lesson of no tie and suit at temple. The older Stephen got, the more beneficial diverse cultures became to my husband and I.

A Diabetic Working Mother

Being a working mother is two tough jobs. The politically correct way to describe mothers who don't have a paying job is to say that they don't work outside of the home. I did a lot of work for my family, "outside of the home" and a lot of Lewis Metal Stamping work "inside of my home." So to say they don't work outside of the home or suggest that working mothers don't do house work isn't exactly correct either. The women without a paying job that I know seem to work continuously. Whether scheduling appointments via cell phone while shopping or decorating or whatever, their work never seems to end. At least on a job outside the home, there is usually a lunch break or a time to commune with others on the job over a sandwich.

Nevertheless, the double duty of an outside job sometimes gets difficult, but it also provides balance in a woman's life. The biggest hindrance to working is not finding time to step back and analyze and summarize issues at home—is my child studying effectively, is my house decorated the way I want it. Are we saving money at the proper rate? Each time that I would get frustrated with the workload of things to do at home and things to do on my paying job; I remember what my dad said to me years ago. I can do anything I want to as long as I'm willing to work hard at it. Further, I remember what my grandfather told me while in high school: some things we simply can't do on our own and we need God's help. It is God's grace that often makes things possible, despite our own efforts. Whenever I get frustrated or think that I can't meet a goal, both my father's and grandfather's words ring loudly in my ears. I take some quiet time to ask God that if it is His will, to please help me, and I'm able to buckle down and put some elbow grease on my work.

Often still today I begin each day by making a list of things that I must get accomplished. It is always a two or three-column list. The lists include 1) things to do at home, 2) errands to run before going home, and 3) things to get done at work. After looking at the list I then prioritize and fit them into my waking hours. They may include: start work early in order to complete a project, or meet a customer, or watch the production flow when I'm not expected to be there; a list of phone calls to make at work, go to the store or pharmacy during my lunch hour, complete analysis, spend staff development time, set up work schedule for tomorrow, get home in time to finish dinner, attend my son's sporting event and bring the team's snack, or take him to Kumon. Accomplishing all of this in a day meant that I had to limit idle chitchat at work or anywhere, set time constraints and plan things efficiently.

As I review my ability to maintain two jobs (at home and at work), I realize that when I am more productive and efficient, I have less time to ponder. When I've been home for a few days due to medical issues and after I've healed, I somehow thought since I had so much time, I would get more done. But the opposite occurred. The more time that I had, the less I actually accomplished. Once I realized that about my ideal work conditions, I had to become disciplined at filling my plate with constructive things to do at an optimal level, not allowing a lull in my work schedule. That discipline took some fine tuning. It is easy to fill your day with busy work; however, it takes discipline to weed out unnecessary or inefficient work. The tasks I chose to do myself have to be the ones crucial to my family and my business and not tasks that others wanted to place in front of me.

When I was trying to sort out how best to spend my time, both at work and at home, I decided that housekeeping chores used a lot of time that I could spend on things that required more concentration and that I enjoyed doing. I decided that what I most disliked and could be done by someone other than me is housecleaning. Housecleaning is much different than designing, decorating and organizing. By housecleaning I mean mopping, vacuuming, dusting, washing and ironing. So I hired a nanny to live in our home. Indeed Joan kept a good handle on that while I was less stressed and had more time to help my son with homework and cook when I felt creative— not daily to feed my family. I had time before she moved into our home to make sure that I created the right environment.

I wanted my son to come home from school by 4 p.m. and not be a "latch key kid," or so I thought. I wanted him to get started on homework early so as not to be rushed at home during the dinner hour. I wanted Joan to feel a welcomed part of our family. And most of all I wanted our house clean and the ironing not to pile up to the point that we felt like we had a new wardrobe when I finally ironed. In essence, what I wanted was a clone to do all of the things that I don't like to do but were necessary.

When we met Joan she introduced herself to all of us with her first and last name. I decided in order to make sure my son always remembered to show respect and so that she felt respected, Stevie and all the kids in our family and the neighborhood called her Miss Joan. On the weekend Joan attended church and went on family outings with us. She cheered at my son's soccer games with the rest of the family. She joked with my husband and once took him down on the kitchen floor and trimmed his toenails because he wouldn't do it himself. We all laughed so hard. She was sick of hearing me complain of his toenails being too long, so she cut them herself.

Joan and I often talked of our similar beliefs on raising children. She even cared for my dog. I have pictures of her playing with my dog in the snow. The pictures are of her rolling around in the snow. I had to remind her that those of us from climates native to snow don't roll around in it.

❀ ❀ ❀

Chapter Three

The Entrepreneur

My Dad – The Entrepreneur

*D*uring my junior year in high school, my father left his job at Ford and became a stamping supplier to the domestic automotive companies. As a parent now, I think back at what a risky move that was just two years before I entered college. Or maybe it wasn't risky for him, just risky for me. My mother also worked at a different division of Ford and during the early years of the business provided family income and medical insurance.

Even as a child I watched as my dad worked long hours, was angry about business losses and elated about business successes. It is still beyond me how my parents were prepared financially to send me to college two years after starting a business and six years after buying five acres of land and building a house there. I don't know why I am so baffled, when I know they were faithful believers in God's ability to make a way out of seemingly no way. I wasn't one of those rich kids at the university whose parents' cash freely covered tuition and other school expenses without sacrifice. I didn't have some education trust account. Nor did I receive any financial aid or take out student loans. My parents saved, and, beyond the grace of God, I don't know how they paid tuition and my living expenses.

Early one morning before going to class, my father asked me to fill in for his secretary. Evidently she didn't show up that morning for work. My father's plant was about 7 miles from campus so I drove to the plant and answered phones, typed and took messages. After two days I received a phone call from the secretary's adult daughter looking for her mother. I explained that she wasn't at work and had not been here the whole week, nor did she call. The daughter hung up and I relayed the details of the call to my dad. Later that day, my father received a call from the same daughter explaining that they found her mother in a hotel room dead from a deadly mix of sleeping pills and alcohol.

After the funeral we learned that the secretary was depressed about personal issues. But what I didn't know was that my dad had been conducting his own little investigation. In many small businesses, besides answering the phone, typing and filing, the secretary also did the office purchasing and bookkeeping for the company. As a regular part of signing checks for bills, my father noticed a higher than usual amount for an office supply company. When the secretary produced the invoice, it included a box of 100 tampons. A small plant in the 1970s had few women and so he questioned her purchase. The secretary explained that she ordered them for personal use, for her and her daughters, and would pay him back. He instructed her not to make personal purchases with company resources and she agreed.

Curious about how many other invoices might include her personal items, he reviewed more vendor invoices. Indeed two tool sets were ordered when only one was required. She promised to pay. Nervous about what other abuses may have occurred, he checked bank statements and cancelled checks. He then browsed the unused check supply and found missing checks. He also reviewed deposit slips and didn't find one for her personal check reimbursing the company for her personal purchases. When she explained that it must have been a bank error, Dad instructed her to reconcile the missing check issue with the bank and not to return until she did. That all happened the week before she went missing.

The bank identified $75,000 in fraudulent checks that the secretary forged. She would cash a petty cash check for the company and cut and forge one for the same amount for herself. My mom could only think of the beautiful wedding the secretary gave her daughter and how Lewis Metal Stamping paid for it. My dad could only remember that while she forged checks, there were often times when he didn't pay himself. I returned to class full time with new found knowledge and my dad began to grow the company, again.

Dad's Heart Attack

At 19, they forced me to graduate from the pediatric endocrinology clinic and I began seeing the same internist that my parents were seeing. I would often ask how my dad was doing medically. My concern was with his heart, especially since he still smoked. My dad was 40 years old when he had his first heart attack. My dad told us that the doctor recommended angioplasty. At that time there were only two institutions in the U.S. that performed angioplasty; the University of Michigan hospital and a hospital in Atlanta. Although the University of Michigan was closer, the waiting list was shorter in Atlanta, so that's where he was in line. While waiting, one night he began to feel chest pain and my mother drove him to the hospital.

Mom later explained that she wasn't about to wait while EMS tried to figure out how to get to our house down our country roads. My mother called me at my apartment. I didn't have my car on campus so my boyfriend's roommate agreed to take me. The emergency room gave my dad nitroglycerin to ease his pain; however, they admitted him to the ICU for further observation. The next morning I took the university bus to the hospital and found my dad asleep with eight IV bags hanging from him. I knew something had happened between the ER visit the night before and his condition the next morning. As I spoke to him, he drifted off to sleep. It was then that the doctors told me that he had a heart attack during the night.

They continued that he was at the best place to have a heart attack—meaning that he had medical staff already there and prepared to save his life. What is so difficult to think about is that angioplasties are now done almost routinely at most hospitals. The angioplasty would have prevented the damage caused by the heart attack.

It's no wonder, however, how Dad developed heart disease. He had a glass bowl ashtray at work that I watched him empty about 3 times during the day because it was too full. After he healed and got back to normal he joked about how badly the paddles hurt. He said the doctors yelled, "Mr. Lewis, Mr. Lewis." He says he answered, "What! . What, would you stop doing that, it hurts!" After his hospital stay, he got so back to normal than he began smoking again. He didn't smoke nearly as much, but he smoked.

Every opportunity that I got I tried to get him to quit smoking. I was at the kitchenette table studying in my apartment and needed a break. But I wasn't exhausted, so I wrote my dad a letter. I'd never written him a letter and somehow it felt good to finally share with him all the things that I'd been thinking. I started out by saying that I admired him and I was proud of the work he does. I told him that I guess I was so proud that I even pick boyfriends who look or act like him. At the end of the letter I gave him a multiple-choice question of why I wrote the letter. I asked whether it was (a) Because my most derelict boyfriend looked most like him, or (b) Because I loved him, or (c) Because I wanted him to stop smoking, or (d) All of the above. I closed with letting him know that it was indeed (d) All of the above.

Losing My Spiritual Mentor

My graduate studies actually began during my senior year of undergrad. So I hadn't yet graduated when my grandfather was again diagnosed with lung cancer. He was first diagnosed with lung cancer when I was in high school.

Surgeons removed his right lung, and there was no more cancer detected. Somehow the cancer had returned and had infected his left and only lung. The prognosis was grim and my grandmother was by his side for radiation treatments. He was tired and couldn't keep his food down. My grandmother bought a juicer hoping that he'd get nutrients from juicing his food. Nothing seemed to work. Finally, the doctor admitted him to the hospital. They gave him oxygen to breathe. He still wasn't getting enough oxygen so they decided to sedate him and put him on a respirator. I remember that he didn't want the respirator in his mouth and tried to fight it. As they wheeled him away to sedate him, he looked at us desperately to stop them. We knew it wasn't something that he wanted, but it was something that the doctors talked us into doing. I will never forget the look he gave us, and despite understanding from the doctors how this would be more comfortable, it hurt me to know that we were doing something that he didn't want.

They sedated my grandfather, so that he wouldn't fight the respirator. He then laid in a coma for almost a month. My grandmother lived with my aunt during that period. My aunt worked at the hospital and brought my grandmother with her every day to sit all day long at the hospital hoping that he'd get better.

After church one Sunday, we went to visit him at the hospital. The doctor wearing green scrubs and a surgeon's cap came out to tell my grandmother and the rest of the family that my grandfather's heart stopped beating earlier in the day. We gasped and he continued that it is the hospital policy that if his heart stops beating again, the doctors won't revive him. I could only imagine his words falling on my grandmother's ears. As hurtful as it was to hear it myself, I could only imagine how piercing it was for my grandmother.

I recall being shocked and angry at the doctor for being so matter of fact about such a grave issue. So I told the doctor as much and told him he was out of line and had no business practicing medicine.

I went into my grandfather's intensive care room and watched the nurses and doctors work on him. I read his chart and saw that his creatinine was high. I knew that creatinine was a measure of kidney function from my diabetes training. The nurse explained that my grandfather's kidneys were failing. His Foley bag barely had urine in it. The doctor, the same one I yelled at, overheard our conversation and asked if I was a nurse. I explained that I wasn't, just diabetic—that's where my medical training came from. From the look on his face, I think he contemplated whether he should even be practicing medicine.

The Sunday evening that the movie "The Last Day" (it was about what life would be like post nuclear war) aired, my mom called to say that they don't think my grandfather would make it through the night. She and my Dad and brother were headed to the hospital to be with my grandmother. It would take too long for me to get from Ann Arbor to Detroit and my car wasn't exactly reliable. So I didn't go. Just as the movie ended, my mother called to say, "He's gone."

I wrote my grandfather's obituary and nervously contemplated how my grandmother would get along without him. They relied completely on one another. My grandfather never cooked and my grandmother never learned to drive. My grandmother always prepared his meals and he always drove her wherever she wanted to go. As a child, I always prayed that if the Lord took one of them He'd take them both. I couldn't imagine one without the other.

When we went to the funeral home to see my grandfather before the funeral, it felt as though there was a hole in my stomach. I was afraid that this would be too much for my grandmother. Although he had been terminally sick for a month, I wasn't prepared for how immensely it hurt. My mother, aunt, cousin, and of course Granny went to the funeral home. As we all stood around the casket looking at him, sniffing and crying silently, my grandmother broke the silence by telling the funeral director that his mouth wasn't done right and his mustache that had overgrown in intensive care, needed trimming. Just then she reached in her purse and pulled out his glasses. She said, "He always wore his glasses," and she positioned them on his face. I couldn't believe how calmly she took all this in and made decisions. Her calmness quieted the rest of our angst.

I remember we had three services for him: a memorial service at the Amherstburg church where he was pastor, a wake at Macedonia Baptist Church in Detroit, where he first became a minister, and then the funeral also at Macedonia. It was hard to go through three services and seeing him in the casket three times. But so many people loved him and it was good for my grandmother to hear how much he was loved. Thea of course came to my grandfather's funeral and met our extended family.

Racial Awakening

When I was in college, there didn't seem to be much outward racial tension. However, minority enrollment decreased from the days of the 1960s BAMN (By Any Means Necessary) movement. The summer between my junior and senior year, I enrolled in a summer program to take classes and look at the graduate school of Public Policy at the University of Michigan. The program was held at member APPAM (Association of Public Policy and Management) schools. In addition to Michigan, they included Harvard, Yale, Minnesota, Stanford, Texas and some others. I applied for admission at what is now known as the Ford School, named after alum and former President, Gerald R. Ford. I was admitted as a Sloan fellow into the accelerated program, which began concurrently with my senior year of undergraduate studies and was completed the following year. I completed all of the prerequisites the first year except for one microeconomics class that I took the summer between graduate school terms. I felt comfortable enough asking one of my female graduate school professors who happened also to be on the admissions committee, why I got into this accelerated program. My grades were decent, but not exceptional; my GRE (Graduate Record Exam) was marginal at best. She explained that they selected students based upon whether they demonstrated success and would be likely to successfully complete the program. She continued that they considered what may have happened if they didn't gain my interest in the program early: they may have lost me to another school. What she didn't further explain was that while our program was diverse in terms of men and women, Christian, Jews, and other religions, there were only two of us who were African-Americans—me and my pal Reggie; and in a public policy studies program, diverse perspectives and ideas are crucial.

Reggie did his undergraduate work at Howard University. Howard University's reputation among many black students was that it graduated black America's elite. Reggie wasn't stuffy or conceited, but he was stylish and always wore designer clothes. Any slacks that weren't blue jeans were dressed up as far as I was concerned. I remember once when Reggie came in late for our economics class. I saved him a seat next to me in the second row. He excused himself and carried his briefcase (not back pack like the rest of us) over other student's heads. The professor, known to be a jokester, held his hand as if to be carrying drinks on a serving tray above his head and said "Oh, Reggie, so glad you could make it, your seat is right here. Barry Manalow will be on soon." I know a professor being a jokester sounds like an oxymoron, but to put in perspective this professor is a well-respected economist.

Reggie and I also took a graduate school class in program management. The professor taught the course from excerpts from the text book that he was writing for the course. The course detailed analytical tools to evaluate the effectiveness of government programs. It was filled with equations for setting up regression analyses and methods of determining the coefficients to be used for each variable. The professor's approach to program management was very quantitative and was a challenge for the entire class. We didn't have many assignments, just a few tests and a final. I remember studying for a test in this class alone in my apartment. I started thinking about how fortunate I was to be in this accelerated program, that it would be cheaper for my parents since I would finish a year earlier than planned. I was getting tired of school, and graduating early sounded good. And then I began to wonder again why I had been accepted to an accelerated program.

Even though the professor explained the benefit to the school, I still felt that the whole diversity thing was to benefit only me or others who look like me. I learned later and with some maturity, that indeed schools can boast high graduation rates when they select students who are most likely to graduate. The diversity benefit to the university and the entire student body was that it created an environment with differing perspectives and exposed all the students to decision making that took into account those differences. It was all so much more than I could completely understand at that time.

Creating a diverse learning environment for the student body, particularly in the public policy field of study, brings several perspectives to policy issues. When students can learn from one another how different perspectives come into play based upon life experiences, the material becomes more tangible and the lessons are better learned than if it were merely lectured and explained hypothetically.

Unfortunately, at that point in my studies I wasn't mature enough to understand the business of higher education, nor did my colleagues in the program. So while trying to study for an exam, my studies were interrupted by thoughts of, "Why do the other students, whether from Long Island, NY or Appalachia, look at me for comments on poverty and federal programs? Why would minimum wage be a concern for me?" Being black doesn't always mean being poor. My parents paid for my education. I began to cry as I pondered these questions—instead of studying. Before I knew it two hours had passed and I hadn't studied anything. I was then mad that this was even an issue, still hindering me from academic excellence.

This was a very perplexing issue for me. I was happy to be in the program, but wondered if in fact, I deserved to be in the accelerated part of it. The professor's perspective was an interesting one and I had never thought of educational institutions as businesses that compete for students likely to succeed, boosting graduation statistics and possibly becoming publicly successful and citing their university for making it possible. The university couldn't boast about its academic performance statistics if students in their program weren't successful. I finally concluded that they admit students who demonstrate evidence of success and possess the skills and qualities that lead to further success. What they do is admit students who contribute to making the student body a diversely woven fabric.

The next day we took the exam and afterwards I felt pretty comfortable about my performance. But you know how that goes, despite how you feel, you could have missed something. So a week later, the professor passed out the graded exams. He handed me mine first and quietly looked me in the eye as I read it. The red note at the top read "A, highest score in the class". I couldn't believe it as I quietly shared it with my friend Reggie. The professor explained that this was a difficult exam and that we should expect lower grades than we're used to. Lower grades; how could that happen if I did well? I left immediately after class. But you know Reggie; he hung around and socialized and no doubt bragged about his friend who blew the curve to hell.

The rest of the class couldn't leave well enough alone; they made sly comments in the program mail room about me ruining the curve in that class. I didn't offer a word. This test and my performance finally proved to me why I belonged where I was. I felt better about my lot in life and at school. I got down on my knees and thanked God not only for the good grade, but for the experience of going through the exercise of understanding my worth. I guess the hard work was to understand my value and what I can expect. However the true lesson was that I was still covered by Jesus' blood and could still count on Him.

College life was busy and I didn't schedule regular appointments with my doctor as my mother had done when I was growing up. I was seen by physicians at the University of Michigan hospital, but at that time I was transitioning between the pediatric and adult clinic.

Because my friends in graduate school were from New Jersey, Washington D.C., North Carolina and St. Louis, the

Easter break was too short a period of time for them to buy airline tickets home. They often came home with me for Easter dinner. We'd load up the leftovers and take them back to school. I bet it made my Dad rethink Boston College and out of state tuition. One Easter they even spent the night at my parents' house so that we could go to Easter sunrise church service at 6 a.m. That was fun, and awful generous of my parents.

Working For Lewis Metal Stamping

My Dad became an entrepreneur when he was 37 years old. Just two years prior, he bought five acres of land and built a house for us to move into the country, away from Henry Ford's Inkster. Inkster is a Detroit suburb located just west of Dearborn, Michigan, Ford Motor Company's home. In the early years of labor unionization, some speculate that Inkster was built to be a city to house the black auto workers brought into the company to thwart unionization efforts. My parents were both employees of Ford Motor Company. As much as I watched and learned from my parents on how to save and run a successful household, I am still amazed when I recount the timing of their decision to build a new house, two years later start a business and in two more years pay for my college tuition. They were the best financial planners I know.

During my last year of graduate school and after interviewing with government agencies like the US General Accounting Office, I thought about how much hard work my dad had done and how wonderful it was that he formed his own business. My father began his career at General Motors as an assembler. He was promoted to supervisor and went to college at night. He moved to a position in Quality Assurance at Ford Motor Company. Shortly before I started college, he took a leave of absence from Ford to become one of its first black-owned automotive suppliers.

As I contemplated my future, I also thought about how my dad and mom had paid (financially and through blood, sweat and tears) for my education and how I wanted to give something back. I thought to myself, if one day I'd like to do my own thing, why not learn from the best: my dad.

I called my dad at work, about a half hour away from school. I asked if I could come to his office and talk to him that Wednesday at 2 p.m. He said, "Sure, but you don't need an appointment to speak with your old man." I quickly said "Ok, Wednesday at 2," and hung up the phone. When I arrived, I had on my gray interviewing suit and white shirt. He looked prepared for me to give him some bad news because I never dressed up for the usual request for cash. After I shook his hand and handed him my resume he took on a whole new posture. I told him I was interested in working for Lewis Metal Stamping and I understood that he was in need of a production control manager. The key to a good interview is to research the company's needs. I had spoken with my mother and of course with her human resources background she knew what his hiring needs were. He said, "Indeed I am," and begun to tell me a little about the position.

So sure enough the Monday after my graduate school graduation I started working at Lewis Metal Stamping. I was a young single woman working for my dad. I felt extra pressure to show that I was hard working and because I worked for my dad, make sure that my conduct was proper for that of the boss's daughter. To any guy appearing as if he wanted to start a personal relationship, I maintained a stiff, strictly business type of demeanor. So I passed on a lot so as not to appear "loose" or "privileged" or "Daddy's Girl". Somehow, I thought people who worked at their father's firm were paid a fat healthy salary for doing nothing. Their degree was not a set of skills but a club membership for Daddy's Firm. What I grew to understand, at least at Lewis Metal Stamping, is that indeed there was no one who worked harder than me and there was no one more privileged to work with James O. Lewis than I was.

With my sheepskin in hand, I thought I knew everything and was ready to take on the world. My father focused my eagerness to sprint my way into my career by explaining that my degrees were like a toolbox. I had a neat little package of tools with instructions, but I had never built anything before. So my value to the firm wouldn't be high until I had built something and gained experience from it. Whenever he explained business and how it works, he always made the point that "some things you learn simply by being on this earth long enough." This clearly explained my lack of a big corporate salary. My initial thought coming in was that I have this master's degree and can help my father to take the company to new heights. As I took on more complicated assignments the more I appreciated my need for experience at using my tools and as my father expected, the more proficient I became at my job. When I reflect on that transition from school to work, I realize that my father didn't stop paying for my education when I graduated from school.

When my dad founded Lewis Metal Stamping in 1978, he was one of the first minority suppliers in the industry. Each of Detroit's Big Three embarked on minority supplier development programs to meet the government's requirement to purchase at least 5% from minority suppliers. In the early 1970s there were no minority supplier companies. In order to meet government purchasing targets, the U.S. automotive manufacturers began to cultivate minority-owned companies from eager would-be entrepreneurs within their companies.

My father was fortunate to have that opportunity with Ford Motor Company. He worked diligently to lease plant space, negotiate and even barter for equipment. The Big Three were growing suppliers from scratch in capital intensive markets, and funding for these companies also had to be developed.

Each of the Big Three worked with its own lending source at "reasonable interest rates". They were Minority Enterprise Small Business Investment Companies (MESBIC). According to the U.S. Small Business Administration, MESBICs are federally funded private venture capital firms licensed by the US Small Business Administration. For these new minority entrepreneurs the prospect of owning their own company was exciting and held promise for what they could do in their own communities. At the same time, because of how capital intensive automotive manufacturing is, these courageous entrepreneurs were leveraged as they had never been before.

While I don't remember all of the business that my parents discussed surrounding this venture, I do recall hearing from my dad later that our home was used as collateral for the initial loan. With a promise of purchase orders from the automakers, a funding source for new business start-ups, it appeared the automotive supply business was going to diversify.

I worked hard to add value to the organization. I joined the company just in time to implement the new computer system. I quickly got to know who was responsible for what at LMS and generally understood their job. The new computer requirements included communicating with the customer electronically to receive part requirements and to send shipping information prior to the shipment arrival. On the accounting end, it was a natural progression to electronically post invoices to the accounting records. The software also maintained shipping and invoice histories. Finally I added some value. In my spare time I represented the company at charity events.

In a small company, implementing a computer system is a side job, the job I was paid to do was customer service. I communicated with customers about any variances in production schedules and hiccups in production. I was a glorified messenger delivering production information to customers. It was stressful listening to customers scream when parts weren't ready when they wanted them. I recall one time listening to a customer from the customer plant that my dad used to work at, scream and cuss at me because we didn't have parts. After we finally appeased him with a date when parts would be shipped, I calmly went to the ladies room and cried my eyes out. I told my dad that I didn't mind being yelled at, but if I was going to take responsibility for not having parts then I needed responsibility and authority for getting parts. He agreed and taught me to schedule the plant.

As I got ready to implement phase II of the computer system which was manufacturing reporting, I learned more about the production end of company. As I better understood what went on in the plant and what needed to happen, I saw a way to improve efficiency. In order to accomplish that level of efficiency, I felt that we needed to improve the skill level in some key manufacturing positions. My uncle worked as shipping manager, making sure that parts were packaged and shipped to customer locations according to the customer's specifications. He did a fine job in the early days when the company was small and the customer locations were few.

Replacing my uncle with a more computer literate employee would be tough, not only for me but for my father as well. Besides him being my elder, he was my uncle. Besides being my father's older brother, he was the very first employee that Lewis Metal Stamping had. It was my father and uncle who started in the early days. My father met with customers, won business, purchased tooling, bought steel and instructed my mother on how to invoice customers. It was my uncle who set dies, made parts, packaged parts, shipped or delivered parts to the customers.

My dad suggested that my uncle look into his retirement benefits and he found that he could afford to quit work. My dad told him not to worry, that somehow we would fill the hole left by him leaving the company and began to make the transition.

I organized our first company retirement party for my uncle. My dad bought him a gold watch with an inscription written on the back. My cousin, on my mother's side became the new production control manager. My uncle's retirement made a way to fill my uncle's position with someone able to manage the computer requirements as well as the shipping schedules.

My father promoted the truck driver, a young energetic man eager to advance in the company. The shipping manager reported to me and between the two of us we manufactured what the customer needed in time for shipment—well, most of the time.

My dad hired my cousin some years before I started with the company. He started as a truck driver, with army training. He was hired initially to get him started as he transitioned from military to civilian life. He showed lots of potential and did much more than the truck driver position required. When I worked with him I found that he picked up concepts quickly and understood how things should be organized. He transported work-in-process, and therefore had to know part numbers and which outside processes were performed to which parts, in addition to knowing the location of the outside processors. Years later, I happened to walk into my dad's office while he was discussing patents with my cousin and the best way to market them.

Evidently my cousin had an idea that he wanted to market on his own. I thought to myself, this certainly isn't company related, why is Daddy wasting time on this. After my cousin left, I told my dad that I thought it was a waste of time for him to discuss my cousin's future business plans. He explained to me that maybe it was a waste, but then again, maybe it wasn't. It was that chance that it wasn't a waste, that he kept his faith in. To take this story full circle, years later, my cousin designed blow molded cups shaped like baseballs, got them manufactured and marketed them to the Detroit Tigers.

My father smoked cigarettes. As mentioned previously, while I was in college he suffered a heart attack before he was able to receive (then a new procedure) angioplasty. Even after a second hospitalization for his heart beating too fast, he started smoking again—this time, not right out in front of us, and he hid it completely from my mom. I decided to let him see how I felt. One day at work, I walked into his office and while he was finishing what he was reading, I lit a cigarette and began to smoke it. Now remember, I'm an adult woman in her 20s and in the mid-1980s we didn't have a smoking policy. I told him that if he was going to kill himself, I would too. As if I was a child, he said in a quiet voice, "Jacquie put that out," and continued his work.

Our production problems had gone on for a while and our major customer at the time was growing tired. We had a string of quality rejections and the customer's purchasing manager came out to talk to my dad about the plan to correct the issues. After hours of reviewing previous issues that had already been corrected, the customer representatives continued to rehash the same issues so as to brow beat him. My dad had been working hard to fix the problems and was tired. I remember when the purchasing manager asked my father what his long term plans were, he lowered his head and said, "I'll probably close the place." I couldn't believe my ears. In all our difficult times, I had never heard my father give up that way. After we finished the meeting and the customers left, I went to my office, called my contact at the customer plant and relayed when parts would arrive and the decisions made during the meeting. To my surprise, my contact had heard that my father might close the business. I sternly told him that under no circumstances would he close it. In fact, we would get through this mess and then grow the business. I decided that the last thing we needed was rumors floating around and that I would nip it in the bud. I asked for the purchasing manager's phone number who had just left our plant. Moments later I called her and began by stating strongly that under no circumstances would we close this business (as if I had some say over that).

She remained calm and said, "Jacquie, your father said that he was going to close it." I told her that indeed he said those words and may have considered it as an option, but with or without her business, we would remain in business. She then decided that it was best that she told me the background that I didn't know.

The purchasing manager explained that she was glad that we weren't going to close the business. It was an important business to her company and it was an important business to her personally. What she told me was that she used to work with my dad and that she and her husband frequently had dinner with my parents. She had been to our house and my parents had been to her house. She said that she recalls when I was a little girl. I told her, "Well, good, I'm glad that we got that rumor cleared up so it wouldn't be spread any further."

She heard the break in my voice from trying to hold back tears and she said, "Sure, no problem, Jacquie."

I allowed myself to get too busy and burned out at work. I was too young to know not to take what customers say personally. But after all, it wasn't just my father's name on the building; it was mine too. I asked my dad if I could work somewhere else for a while. He of course allowed me that freedom. I went to work for the US General Accounting Office.

Being hired there was interesting because when I interviewed with the agency on campus, the two up and coming white male GAO recruiters didn't appear interested. But when I sent a letter and resume, the recruiter was very interested. Based upon my letter I interviewed with two people in the office and I was hired, pending an interview with the director.

I came back to meet with him and given my background and training he said that I would feel ahead of the game, and he welcomed me aboard. As if I thought I wasn't making much at Lewis Metal Stamping, I took a $2000 pay cut to take that job and planned to rely on periodic pay increases.

I left for training in Washington D.C for two weeks. Just prior to leaving, my father had an episode of arrhythmia, which means that his heart rate accelerated and didn't regulate until after doctors gave him a shock. The doctors decided to run tests to see which medicines would best control his heartbeat. To do this, he was slightly sedated while they used probes to race his heart and tested different medications to regulate it. While I was in Washington, my father and I arranged to be available by phone and everyone at GAO understood that if I were too concerned about my father's health, I would come home. I spoke with him daily and felt comfortable that he would be ok.

While at GAO, my father talked me into not wasting money on apartments; that a better investment would be for me to buy a house. When I explained that I didn't have money for a down payment, he suggested I move home to save money. So I moved home with my parents to save money, paid my parents $250 a month rent, and with a gift from my grandmother bought my first home. The first week after I moved into my three-bedroom bungalow, someone broke into it while I was at work. When I stepped up on the porch and got ready to put my key in the door. I noticed that the door was standing wide open. I became frightened thinking that perhaps they were still in the house. This was before the days of commonplace cell phones. Despite the fact that this wasn't the way I wanted to meet the neighbors, I went next door to call the police. I explained what happened and we called the police. While waiting for the police, my neighbor interviewed me to understand that I was a single woman, without children.

She was concerned that I was a woman living alone. She and her husband were in their 70s and perhaps he was closer to 80. The husband was impatient with the police and decided to check it out himself. I pleaded with him that it wasn't necessary; the police would be there soon. He insisted. His wife pleaded with him and thought it safer if he waited. He showed us a pistol hidden behind his hand in his pocket and said he'd be safe. He looked in to make sure that no one was still in robbing the place. He returned home to put up his gun just in time for the police to arrive. The robbers were obviously young since most of what they stole was jeans and jewelry and left my business suits. I spent the night at my parents' house, but my father insisted that I spend the next night (after the locksmith changed the locks) at my own house.

My first order of business was to put an alarm on the house. While the installers were working I found an ad for discounted puppies at a pet shop. I thought, "Good, I'll feel safe with an alarm and especially if I get a big dog. When I arrived at the pet store, all of the puppies in sight were small breeds. I asked the attendant if she had any larger breeds.

She had some, but they were in the back room. When she brought them out, they were a brother and sister German Shepard mix. I bought the male, food, collar and a leash for $29.99. I named him Max after the dog in Dr. Seuss' "The Grinch who Stole Christmas."

As I worked at GAO, my father listened at the dinner table to me complain about the slow nature of the work to make sure of its accuracy. He'd ask what I did that day and I sarcastically told him that I stapled and collated. When I had research to copy I told him that I learned to operate a new machine that day, the copier. The work was purposely slow and methodical and I didn't feel like I affected anything.

At the same time, at LMS, my dad had a big contract with General Motors to manufacture the recall portion of a production component and package it for the dealers. He needed reliable support and based on my boredom, asked me to come back. I was delighted, except it would cost him more this time.

My first assignment was to correct the Material Requirements Planning module of the computer system since the job was going into production soon. I noticed that we had a bottleneck in responding to requests for quotes from customers. I watched the process and found that unnecessary time was spent doing cost calculations manually by calculator.

In addition, as I looked for copies of old quotes to verify component cost, the quote sheet was either missing or handwritten and in poor condition. So, before I became busy I spent time developing a quote program that allowed us to spend more concentrated time on the engineering of the part and let the computer do the calculations. After about six month's time, I wrote a quoting program that did all of the same calculations automatically rather than with a calculator.

It also forced us to consistently calculate machine burden rates and administrative costs. I took executive management courses that helped me better understand finance and accounting.

The program worked, was accurate and would use a consistent pricing formula. The program also calculated production rates based on the speed of the press, an allowance for breaks and coil changes. Labor and machine burden rates were based upon those production rates. I tested the program against my father's written notes and calculations and they matched. But I knew it was going to be a tough sell to my father to suggest transitioning to the program. I showed him that I came up with the same prices and let him take the interactive program for a test drive to determine user friendliness and consistent accuracy. Because the program generated three reports: a formal letter to the buyer, a cost sheet for the file (which looked exactly like the manual form), and a cost breakdown for the buyer, it was no longer necessary for the secretary to type handwritten quotes before submitting them to the buyer. My dad approved the program's use but kept a careful eye out for mistakes and spot-checked some quotes using his handy calculator.

What I began to notice was that my dad and I had the perfect relationship. American society makes it natural for daughters to work for their fathers. In father-son relationships, which you see more commonly in business, it can become competitive at some point if the son tries to become the alpha wolf. He challenges the father and wants to prove himself. In mother-daughter relationships a similar situation occurs, except more in the form of who has more influence and who does it better until ultimately a cat fight occurs.

In mother-son relationships the mother can be so busy mothering that her son isn't allowed room to grow. But in a father-daughter relationship, the father pushes the daughter to be aggressive and the daughter understands that he is the boss. As a girl, my mother socialized me to be the one who made sure nothing was undone or forgotten. So to support my dad in business, no matter what was needed, I felt my role was to make sure nothing was forgotten. I always took notes at meetings and reminded him of the deliverables we promised and who was responsible. I also cleaned and organized his office the way I knew my mother would do it. Some of it he liked, some of it he felt was a nuisance. The only time our relationship became difficult was when I was looking for praise or recognition. Because he was my father, I expected it. But when I rethink it, perhaps what I did wasn't that great and didn't deserve the praise I somehow thought it deserved.

Soup Du Jour–
The Automotive Minority Supplier Joint Venture

My father created Lewis Metal Stamping in a very traditional way that many small businesses are established. However, as the domestic auto industry matured and advanced technologically, the Big Three had a need for larger suppliers that could fold into their capabilities manufacturing component systems, performing research and design as well as managing other component suppliers. Having the capability to do these things didn't just mean having the knowledge, but having the resources. Having the resources meant having the sales contracts in order to receive revenue. And so the automotive supply industry began evolving to meet these needs.

Part of what made up the domestic automotive supply base was the competing interests of minority-owned suppliers, the interests of medium-sized white-owned suppliers and how the banks influenced those relationships. The constraints placed by the automakers were complex. The Big Three continued to struggle to meet the government's goal of buying 5% of its material purchases from minority-owned businesses. Even by requiring that large system suppliers purchase 5% from minority-owned suppliers, the targets were not being met. The automakers were concerned about meeting the government's requirement because the auto companies were also suppliers to the government. A concern from a marketing standpoint was the ethnic minority customers that bought their vehicles. The question among leaders in minority communities was why should we buy a vehicle from automakers that don't buy components or do business with companies owned by our community and located in our community, and that employ our community members?

The automakers needed to ensure that its suppliers were financially stable companies and could ensure a constant supply of components without interruption. As more and more suppliers entered the marketplace—both minority and non-minority, it became necessary for the automakers to streamline the supply base thereby limiting the number of companies in the supplier arena.

The minority suppliers were all young companies suffering the corporate growing pains that all young companies suffer. Many of them were formed in the late 1970s and early 1980s. Seed capital secured by the MESBICs was just enough to lease a building and buy used equipment. Even the used equipment was sometimes acquired by bartering services. For instance, my father got some of his plant support equipment by getting the equipment owner an introduction to his customers. Because of the capital requirements, there were very few resources remaining to use as working capital. Working capital is money that the company can use for start up costs necessary to fund new projects.

When a company is growing, these start up cost requirements are typically more than the profit a company receives from its existing business. It is only the profit portion of the selling price that would fund new business projects, since the rest of the selling price pays for labor, materials overhead, and administrative costs of what was sold. Without access to additional money or lines of credit with the banks, the company then uses funds that would otherwise pay for items used in existing production for the new project costs.

So when it comes time to pay the raw material vendor, there is not enough money to do that. This is the start of negative cash flow. Negative cash flow is when the demand for cash (cash required for the purchase of business materials) exceeds the supply of cash (cash coming in from selling current production).

In order to satisfy the negative cash flow, companies attempt to secure additional loans. Many companies go through this same scenario. However when minority-owned companies do it, there is the added hue of racism that adds the often unfounded cloud that the business owners don't understand good business practices. These minority companies were so debt ridden when they were formed that it was hard for them to be strong candidates for additional funding or as long term players in the supply base.

Others in the supply base (non-minority owned companies) were being affected as well when auto companies realized there were too many total suppliers for them to manage. So they began reducing the number of suppliers. Large white-owned companies had technological strong holds in the market which secured their place in the supply base. They were also large companies that could cash flow the large investment required to finance start up cost such as engineering, tooling and start up material. Medium and small white-owned suppliers were at risk of elimination from the automotive supply base.

The fourth player of primary influence in this equation is the banks. In the mid-1980s the domestic auto industry was strong and commercial banking was relatively pleasant. If the big three issued a purchase order, it could be presented to a bank by a supplier and almost work as a promissory note to repay the loan, and the purchase order was sufficient collateral.

I can remember the days when a telephone call from an automaker's buyer would be enough to tip the scales in our favor with the bank's loan committee's decision. Unfortunately, the indebtedness of the minority owned companies while trying to buy equipment and support operations, made additional lending for new programs difficult for the banks to justify.

Therefore, based upon the needs of the automaker to populate its supply base with a limited number of financially viable companies which include minority suppliers; the bank's need to make loans to financially stable companies; the medium-sized white-owned suppliers need for a reason to remain in the supply base; and the minority-owned company's desire to remain in business, the industry was ripe for a perfect storm. And from this condition, the automotive minority supplier joint venture was born.

My definition of the automotive minority supplier joint venture is a business whereby 51% of the corporate stock is owned by an ethnic minority individual or individuals. Forty-nine percent is typically owed by a medium-sized white-owned company. What this ownership structure provided is additional capital for the minority-owned company; a perceived "safe" avenue for the automaker to make the 5% purchases; a place in the supply base for the medium-sized white-owned company to have a marketing edge, and a perceived secure loan for the bank. The reason that this arrangement works for a medium-sized white-owned firm and not another small white-owned firm or a large white-owned firm is because another small firm wouldn't have the financial means to participate, and the large white-owned firm doesn't need the marketing edge in order to remain in the supply base.

The subtle nuances of minority supplier joint venture, while it seemed to be the best thing since sliced bread to the automakers, bank, white-owned firm and chosen minority, reeked of some familiar racist components. A stock ownership split of 51%-49% should yield the same split in profits after expenses. However in many cases when the stock is purchased, the white-owned company may provide as much as 80%-90% of the capital and the ethnic minority brings his or her modest capital, ethnicity and therefore perceived access to customers. Somehow the structure that is formed must be reported (in order to qualify as minority purchases for the automaker) as a 51% minority ownership.

In order for the white-owned firm to benefit from the over-investment in capital, the joint venture finds creative ways for the white-owned firm to be compensated. One way is that profits were not necessarily divided commensurate with the 51-49% ownership split. Profits could be divided according to capital investment instead. Another way for the white-owned company to earn on its underreported capital investment is to charge fees for services or the use of technology that the minority company wouldn't have if not for the joint venture. These fees would be paid from the operating expense of the minority joint venture and taken out before profits were reported.

From the bank's perspective, the white partner (who likely has more significant assets and a banking relationship) has a vested interest in seeing the joint venture's success. The customers find it acceptable because the entity not only has perceived technical and organizational know-how, but bank support. Finally, the majority or white partner is willing to get involved because as the numbers of suppliers decrease, being designated a minority-owned firm seemed to be a way to stay in the game for many medium sized white firms. It became their marketing edge.

The birth of these minority supplier joint ventures began the demise of the legitimately formed minority-owned suppliers. The original minority suppliers that were created from personal savings, extended family savings and using homes as bank collateral and were highly leveraged, were no longer viable in the customer's eye. Minority joint ventures rarely employed ethnic minority employees. Therefore, if through some shell game of stock ownership, automakers were able to meet purchasing targets of 5% through these minority joint ventures, they were not meeting the objective of doing business with companies that employed, paid taxes, and generated wealth in ethnic minority communities. Clearly that was an objective in words, not deeds.

Several minority supplier joint ventures sprung up. The day of starting a business from scratch was over. The days of a company being owned and operated by minority individuals and of ethnic minorities being the true beneficiaries of the firm were dwindling. As a small supplier, without the financial and technical help that these joint ventures brought to the customer, the economy looked bleak for Lewis Metal Stamping.

Developing Peak Performance Blood Sugar Levels

The Impact of Emotions on Diabetes

One of the most important things that I have learned being a diabetic for over 30 years is that blood sugar level played an important role in my ability or inability to work at peak efficiency. I found that if my blood sugar was 250 or higher, I was tired and not a sharp thinker. My energy level was low and it was difficult to get work done. On the other extreme, if my blood sugar was low, I was nervous, jittery almost disoriented and had trouble speaking clearly and coherently.

What that translated into was that if I could not bring my blood sugar to absolutely normal range (70 to 120, or not higher than 150), I had to make sure that my blood sugar wouldn't adversely affect my performance. For instance, when I had speaking engagements or important meetings that relied on my ability to speak clearly and coherently, I made sure that my blood sugar was never low and erred on it being a little high. On the other hand, if I had lots of work to get accomplished or a number of errands to complete during the day, I made sure that my blood sugar wasn't too high, which would zap my energy level.

I remember scheduling a periodic 7am staff meeting so that we could huddle and plot strategy before phones started ringing and customers started making demands. My blood sugar was low and as I tried to conduct the meeting I had to apologize and leave to eat some sugar wafers before finishing the meeting. Likewise when it was high and I had to prepare for a customer presentation the next day. I couldn't do it. Although it was a routine presentation, I needed to customize it for that customer and I didn't have the energy. I waited until the next morning and with normal blood sugar and fresh ideas, I completed the presentation and made copies at home.

Home office equipment was also a necessary part of efficiently running the business with diabetes and being a working mom. There are some times when work has to be done at a place where you can best manage them all, the workload, the diabetes and being a mom. I had extra medication and all the support supplies for my diabetes at work and a computer, fax and copier at home. That's the only way I could effectively be a working mother who owns a company, with diabetes and is sane—well, for the most part sane.

My father always told me that any question could be broken down and analyzed mathematically. Therefore by measuring activity level, insulin level and food consumption, normally I could balance my blood sugar. This fine balance of course required some planning before each upcoming day. I had to plan meals and at all times make sure I had access to emergency food. I kept sugar wafers in my purse, car, desk at work, kitchen and bedroom night stand so that I never had to travel far to cure an insulin reaction. I kept insulin and syringes as well as a spare glucometer to measure my blood sugar at work.

A Moving Corporate Yard Stick

Lewis Metal Stamping had gone through many automotive programs that weren't only a measure of meeting quality, cost, delivery, or technology standards, but were a measure of a company's patience, endurance and resources. Every meeting that introduced the newest requirement to do business became another excuse not to award business to a minority supplier.

If it were the matter of meeting a consistent set of standards that the company either met or didn't meet, that would be ok. But each of the Big Three had its own requirements which allowed the auditor (customer employed) to use his or her own discretion as to whether a supplier met the objectives or not. Certainly as the industry evolved and improved, more stringent standards were applied, but the results of the supplier selection process seemed to suggest that if the auto manufacturer wanted the minority supplier in the supply base, that supplier would marginally pass the audit. If the customer didn't want the company in the supply base, the supplier company would (according to the audit results) not meet the minimum requirements. The marginal score of the suppler that passed the audit allowed the customer to award new business, but easily supported removing the business if the company failed to comply—or it was perceived to fail to comply.

My dad and I went to a customer meeting to listen to the Director of Minority Business (employed by the customer to "manage" the group of ethnic minority suppliers) roll out the customer's latest requirement. We listened with some cynicism; nevertheless we listened to the new set of requirements carefully. It was usually me who lost patience with the whole process, like the time a purchasing manager kept changing the requirement for us to be awarded new business. I lost patience with her changing the parameters and insisted that she commit not to change them for our next meeting. She begrudgingly agreed and left our plant, located in the heart of "the hood." Just outside was a former employee who looked to be a little drunk. She held on to her manager (a black man) to make sure the drunken former employee didn't try to touch her. I peered out the window and laughed and was never happier to see him. My father chuckled while saying, "That's not funny."

After she left, I asked the former employee in to make sure he was ok. He told me, he didn't need my sympathy, "because sympathy was found in the dictionary between shit and syphilis." After he left, I thought about it, and indeed alphabetically he was right. Far be it for me to be between shit and syphilis.

Back to the Minority Director's meeting, my dad became impatient with the moving yardstick of requirements to do business, and each customer had its own version. This particular director was short in stature and wore an outdated jheri curl hair style. A friend of mine and I referred to him as "Jheri Curl." I don't remember what exactly was said, but my father lashed out at the director and told the director that he (the director) didn't have a clue what it took to run a business and meet the ever-changing standards that don't seem to improve the product, just cost more money for the supplier to implement. I couldn't believe my eyes and ears. My father was so right, but I couldn't believe he was telling the director and not just me. The meeting regained its level of composure and ended.

The next day at work, Dad told me that he would call the director to apologize. We agreed that what he said was correct (even other customer managers agreed that it was warranted), but Dad said that his actions could hurt the company. Dad explained that what he said in the meeting was true, but the way he said it didn't show respect for the director's position— whether he thought the director, the man, was worthy of respect or not.

❀ ❀ ❀

Chapter Four

From Tragedy to Triumph

A Hurt Like No Other

I worked for my dad for eight years. I felt like I understood most things, but knew that I didn't know everything. I couldn't have asked for a better supervisor than my Daddy. He knew he could trust me to hold his confidence and have the company's best interest at heart always. With that trust came the responsibility to make a difference. He allowed me to see things as they really were so that I would understand what worked and what didn't work. Part of what the Minority Business Director wanted was a business plan.

The customer wanted to understand the company—where it has been, where it is now, and where we see it in five years. The business plan was due on the upcoming Friday.

On Tuesday my dad decided to stay late and finish the history section of the business plan. My assignment from my dad was to complete the future part of the plan. I understood how my father wanted to grow the business, plus I had ideas, too. I enjoy writing, so I knew it wouldn't take me long. As the work day came to a close, I tried to convince him to call it a day with me, but he decided to stay and finish his portion of the plan.

When I got almost home, my dad called my cell phone. I thought maybe he changed his mind and was going to come visit my son Stevie. He told me that I left my office keys and that he would put them in the top right drawer of my desk.

When I got home, I ran bath water for my son. The phone rang, as I got ready to put him into the water. Steve answered the phone and said that Alice, then my brother Jeff's girlfriend, now his wife, was on the phone. I started to ask if I could call back, but something told me to wait and take the call. So I pulled my son out of the bath water and by the time I got the phone, my mother was on the line. She told me that my father passed out and EMS was on the way. I asked if he was conscious and she said no. I quickly grabbed the diaper bag, slipped clothes on my son and told my husband to get into the car. I drove to my mother's house. My father lay on the floor as EMS workers tried to get a heartbeat. My mother, Jeff, Alice, Steve and I stood there watching and praying for a heartbeat. My husband watched and listened to them call out blood pressure and heart monitor readings until Steve could take it no more. He went across the hall into an unlit office and began to cry with his head in his hands. I was so annoyed that his gesture seemed to give up on my dad. But I didn't have time to deal with that.

Finally they got a heartbeat and transported him to the emergency room. My mother rode in the ambulance and we followed quickly behind them in my car and my brother in his car. When we finally reached the hospital, the admitting nurse didn't ask us to wait in the regular waiting room, but instead asked us to go into a family waiting room by ourselves. Steve had called a cardiologist friend of his to meet us at the hospital, and he did. Shortly after we entered the room a nurse told us that they had lost the heart beat again in the ambulance, but they had one more thing to try and they would continue trying. Moments later, the doctor that Steve called walked in and shook his head in a "no" motion to Steve. A nurse with the hospital chaplain then arrived to tell us that he didn't make it.

In a state of shock, I watched as everyone cried. My son looked around the room at everyone crying and began to laugh. At 18 months old, he didn't understand that we weren't playing "fake cry" with him. Once again, I felt a hole in my heart—a tremendous hole—a hole that was more than an emotional pain, but a very physical pain piercing my chest.

I then began to imagine how hurt my mother was. I looked at my brother, my dad's only son, and could only imagine his sorrow. But the loss I couldn't bear was to know that my son wouldn't remember his grandfather. His grandfather who couldn't wait until Stevie turned "the terrible twos;" his grandfather who used to sing Unchained Melody to me when I was a little girl to fall asleep and when I called him to ask how many stanzas of "Oh My Love" (as Jeff and I called it) do I have to sing before Stevie stops crying and goes to sleep, he drove over to my house and said I probably didn't know all of the words, grabbed Stevie and begun to sing. And Stevie went to sleep.

The nurse asked us if we wanted to see my father. We answered yes and went into the room. I stroked his peaceful forehead and recalled asking Mom if she wanted to kiss him goodbye. I remembered my mom telling me that my grandmother kissed my grandfather after he died. I wasn't there, but I kept the memory of what that must have been like. I turned away as she said her goodbye.

I shook the emotional cobwebs from my head as we left the hospital and began to think of what comes next. We took my mom home in our car and called Lillian Granny from the car phone. My brother picked her up and brought her to stay with my mom. My father passed out at about 7 p.m. in the evening.

We got home from the hospital about the time the 11 o'clock news was on. I know because we turned the television on by habit and that's what was on. While the TV played its role as background noise, we called my dad's sisters who lived about 45 minutes away. Well, really only 30 minutes if they drove on the freeways. But they don't use freeways, so 45 minutes it was. They were naturally devastated to find out that their baby brother and uncle had died. They traveled with my cousins to my mom's house and stayed until past 3 a.m.

They all told their favorite stories about my dad and I told my dad's sister that he had just told an employee about her and the time she baby-sat him and fed him oatmeal with gravy. She said that my dad made the oatmeal and gravy story up, but he was adamant that she made gravy with her oatmeal and served it for dinner. It was nice to have some humor even if it was 3 am and the end of such a tragic evening,

Morning brought my most difficult professional and personal task ever. I had to relay the tragedy to the employees at Lewis Metal Stamping. After spending the night at my mom's house with my husband, son, and brother, I called ahead to have our administrative assistant assemble all of the managers along with the entire plant in the plant meeting room. As I arrived to the plant, I drove past the building because I could see some stragglers still moving toward the meeting area. Finally I went in. I planned to remain professional while I explained to people that my father died suddenly last night and they would continue to have a job and they shouldn't worry as we went forward. It didn't exactly work that way. As I walked in, the administrative assistant asked, "Do you know where Mr. Lewis is? I've been trying to reach him to give him a message." That was very unlike my father as he was always in the office early unless he had a meeting off site and the administrative assistant would have known that. I appeared preoccupied and went directly to the meeting area. She followed. I thought the best thing to do was to be direct and come straight out with it. "Mr. Lewis had a heart attack and died last night," I said. As strong as I tried to be, I couldn't hold back the tears. A supervisor grabbed me and I cried into his chest. The plant manager asked that we bow our heads in prayer. He led us in prayer and then got everyone back to work.

I spent the rest of the day sitting in my dad's office thinking about all of the memories, how much I loved him, how much he loved me. I sat uncomfortably in his office trying to imagine what he would tell me to do. I just wanted to hear his voice, lay my head on his chest while he hugged me as he had done so many times before. Eventually I snapped out of it and made sure that there wasn't anything on his desk that was pressing and required immediate attention. I was amazed that I was aware of most of what needed to be done. Nothing caught me by surprise. I went through his phone messages and the papers on his desk. I instructed the administrative assistant to tell any of his callers that he wasn't in, and ask if someone else could help. If not, take a message and I would return the call later. Everything seemed surprisingly "handled." Nothing required my immediate attention. Almost as if my dad had planned for a quiet day for me, I had lots of time to think about what the implications of him not being at the company anymore meant. I had time to think about him not being in my life anymore and how I would need to keep his memory alive for my son to know who he was. That fact troubled me most. Later that evening, our attorney met us at the plant to discuss what legal matters we would need to handle.

I couldn't help but recall what my dad said when I told him Steve and I were serious about one another. He asked me, "What can Steve get me? At least the other guy had access to baseball tickets." Well, I guess Steve did give him a nice funeral. One benefit of being married to a funeral director is that I will never go to a funeral home to pick out a casket and plan a funeral service. If by chance Steve predeceases me, my son's godmother, also a funeral director, will arrange it. Steve met with my mother at her house to finalize the recommendations he made. Steve was unable to embalm my father because they were too close. Our friend, my son's godfather, and another funeral director embalmed him.

When it came time to view my father's body for the first time, I came from the plant and met my mother and brother at the funeral home. My husband wasn't there and I purposely got there early, before the time I told my mother. I knew that the initial shock of seeing him dead and in the casket would be tough to deal with. I wanted to be strong for my mother and brother so I got there early to prepare.

His body was laid out in an alcove with some of the flower arrangements sent early. I looked at him and had the urge to nestle my head into his chest. It's amazing how important a hug is—the whole experience—the brush of his wool suit, his smell, the brush of his chin on my forehead, a grunt or hum. When you hug someone, each person has their own unique way of holding and shrugging their arms. Months later I went into his closet, hoping his scent was still there, but it wasn't.

As we walked into the church before the funeral to view my father for the last time, I put his calculator, a mechanical pencil and some 3" X 5" cards in his front jacket pocket. You'd never find my dad without his calculator and a mechanical pencil. Even on the weekend when he didn't have on a suit coat, he'd clip a mechanical pencil to the neck of his pullover shirt. If God had a mathematical question, my dad would be lost without his supplies. I don't really believe that, but somehow it felt good to do. In a way, I didn't want to see his calculator lying around unused. And I couldn't bring myself to throw it away.

At the service, lots of family and friends were there. Of course, business associates and flower arrangements from business associates flooded the church. So many friends and business colleagues told stories of how he made a difference in their lives. During the service the minister asked those offering words to hold their comments to two minutes. I had heard ministers do this before and understood that it was so that the service didn't hold too long and so that the family wasn't put through undue strain. But I remember listening to what so many had to say and I knew there were more. I felt like I could sit there for another hour listening.

After the service, I saw my dad's old co-worker from Ford, the family that we used to visit when I was a little girl. He had suffered two heart attacks of his own and my dad helped him and his wife during that time. His wife was talking to my mother and when I walked over she grabbed her husband who was sobbing. She explained that he was so upset that he was unable to speak. As I watched this adult man stricken by grief, I realized that our family wasn't alone in deep loss.

Lewis Metal Stamping – On My Own?

For the next several months, I conducted business as if my dad was on vacation. In fact I told the staff that they should treat reporting systems as if he were on vacation. For the most part that worked, for a while.

As a normal part of their process, the bank asked me to submit a transition plan. It was good because it required me to think step by step about what needed to be done and how I would operate without my dad's skill set. It also forced me to figure out who I needed to convince of what. In addition to the bank, there were vendors with large account balances who were critical to production flow that I had to convince that the business would continue. At the same time as handling the bank and major vendors I went on a marketing crusade to contact customers and convince them that I could and would run the business. I felt as though I had a small window of time whereby customers would be sympathetic and at least hear my plan of continuation. In many cases, customers were eager to help, but not in the case of one. This purchasing representative allowed me to schedule a meeting with him only to restate his decision to eliminate Lewis Metal Stamping from his supply base. It was hard to believe that both my parents once worked with this man.

Grief has a physical impact on the body as well as an emotional impact. I know for me, it seemed grief alone, independent of what I ate, caused my blood sugar to rise. The ultimate effect it had on my body was that I lost weight. The grief of losing my father made me disinterested in eating. However it is critical that diabetics taking insulin eat to maintain normal blood sugar levels. I continued to take my normal dose of insulin, however I didn't eat much and I didn't suffer from insulin reactions. The human body is for the most part a self healing system—when we have infections, white blood cells rush in to fight the infection. Likewise, when my blood sugar became dangerously low my liver secreted glucose as an emergency backup for when I wasn't eating. By not consuming calories, the result was that I lost some weight.

The sting of losing my father caused a pain in my chest, a pressure that wouldn't go away no matter what I did. I can remember thinking when will this pain end? When will life go back to normal? Of course life never goes back to what we remember as "normal", but what happened over about a six month period of time was that I first learned to work through the pain and later learned how to suppress the pain and turn it into joyous memories of my father that I could draw upon as life lessons.

I should have expected there to be some turnover in staff, but I didn't. I envisioned that everyone would rally around me to make the company successful. But my lack of experience caused me not to plan for that event. There were some who immediately left and others who took longer to find other jobs. At 31 years old, I took the turnover personally. For many, it was too much a gamble to entrust their family's livelihood to a 31 year old woman. For employees with no dependent family or with adult children, or with faith in my ability, that was a risk they could take.

The month immediately following my father's death the balloon payment on the mortgage for one of the buildings came due. This was something I never worked on with my father. I certainly met our bank loan officer; however, my father typically handled the banking relationship. So I relied on the education that my parents invested in me to settle this issue.

The company's sales were suffering, making cash flow tight. The debt load and resulting balance sheet were not healthy and therefore made refinancing this balloon difficult. The bank that originally held the note never said they would not refinance it, however my mom and I felt the bank's rate was too high. Besides, the bank's attitude throughout the process made us feel as if we didn't deserve this business. After all, who ever heard of two women trying to run a manufacturing company? Two black women no less! So we shopped the mortgage at other banks. My mother (Chairman, who inherited my father's shares of the business) and I (President/CEO) visited bank after bank to try to refinance the mortgage.

The company's financial situation was difficult enough, but combining the hurt of losing my father with rejections from bank after bank was salt in our wounds. We made attempts at several local banks and was even introduced to one local bank's loan committee by a friend of ours who worked at the bank. All of our attempts yielded negative responses. Not only did they not offer a competitive interest rate, but they did not want to take over the mortgage at any rate. It seemed that our quest to find a better interest rate had to be refocused to finding a bank that would finance the note, given our recent string of financial losses. Finally we decided that despite how terrible we were treated at the bank that held the original note, we could at least get financed.

When my father purchased the buildings, he did so personally and leased them to the business. Therefore the buildings were now owned by my mother. Angry about how we were treated, I gathered my mother's loan documents and reviewed the payment amount. The documents were written such that the note would need to be negotiated again in five years. There was no penalty for prepayment, so I decided that we would never have to refinance a balloon again. I calculated a depreciation schedule that would pay enough principle each month so that the building would be paid off in five years rather than 15. I made my own payment coupons for my mother to use when paying the note. Along with our attorney we drew up a lease agreement between my mother and Lewis Metal Stamping at an increased lease note so that she could pay additional principle and repay the loan before it needed to be renegotiated. Lewis Metal Stamping paid my mother increased rent and she in turn paid the bank the increased mortgage payments that I put on the new payment coupons.

Indeed, the building was paid off in five years and we never had to refinance a balloon, ever. The exercise in calculating a payment amount that would pay off the loan in a specific number of payments at the given interest rate validated my education and was a real life application that proved that the formulas I learned in school really do work.

Besides my baptism by fire of fixed asset financing, I probably spent the first couple years of running the company making safe decisions that didn't hurt the business and kept it going, but didn't grow the business. When my father died, Lewis Metal Stamping was experiencing tight cash flow and was in a vulnerable position with customers. I was concerned how the banks' long arms may impact my mother personally and so I took steps to untie her personally from the business and offer myself to the wolves at the bank instead. I ran the business very meagerly and didn't adjust my salary because I had limited personal resources to float a payroll from my pocket like my father had done.

From the Wednesday morning after my father died, and for the next six months, I worked at a rapid and steady pace that I had never worked at before. I understood why the bank, customers, suppliers and employees required so much of me.

I also knew that no one other than me could provide them with what they wanted. In addition to refinancing the balloon on the plant mortgage, I had to visit with customers to assure them that the company would continue to manufacture product for them; assure suppliers that they would get paid; and assure employees that they would have a means to feed their families. For the most part, customers understood my purpose in meeting with them. However what most of them didn't understand was that it was difficult personally to talk about my father and the future of the business he founded and I would continue to run without him. Because I was on a road show of explaining to the world what my continuation plan was, I structured all my presentations to go into the meeting, be cordial, and stick to the facts of the matter—the company needed new business in order to grow, and to be a good supplier it needed to grow exponentially. The only way that I could get through these presentations was to limit my emotional involvement. I could manage quick condolences, but not extended conversation about my dad. No customer understood what I was going through except one, Sandy.

Sandy greeted me in her office lobby. She made no small talk as we walked down the hall to her office. Before I sat down and began to explain how the company would continue, she stopped me and explained how difficult it was to lose her father. She continued that for months, if not years, she couldn't even say his name. As my iced over façade and game face began to melt, tears filled my eyes. At first I was upset that she broke through my way of dealing with this phase of my life, but as we talked about my dad and his work, I appreciated being able to break down, and remember that I was not just an operations manager who lost her boss, but a daughter who lost her father, with a son who will never know his grandfather.

Finally, years of reducing expenses and heavy marketing began to bare fruit. I finally moved my belongings into my father's office and began to accept the fact that I had to run this company and stop coasting. Once I borrowed money from my mom for two days to float a payroll. I vowed from then on, I would never be in that position again. The payroll liability was moved to the beginning of the week so that if something didn't make the cut, it wouldn't be payroll. We even decided to spruce up the office. We painted and replaced some carpeting and I painted my dad's office pale pink. It was conservative beige with brown wood furniture when he was there. I had the walls painted a pale pink and bought a cherry desk and hutch. With those modest changes, it began to feel like my own. My brother joked, "Dad would roll over in his grave to know you painted his office pink!"

I also bought conference room chairs and a new station for our administrative assistant to greet visitors without them peering onto confidential documents on her desk. I felt that in order for me, a young, black female manufacturing CEO, to be taken seriously, I needed my own professional look. The company needed a more professional look. New digs do give you a new attitude. We hosted customer presentations in our new conference room and even developed a new brochure.

We began to get new business from new customers. The Big Three were now requiring that their large system suppliers purchase 5% from minority businesses. The new growth and booked sales should have been a 60% increase in sales if managed properly. While we had equipment and resources in place, what I missed in that equation was that we didn't quite have all of the right people in place. As we began to launch the new parts, scheduling, quality, and cash flow issues started to arise. With the right skill set, quality and scheduling issues wouldn't have occurred. Scrap and the downtime of scheduling problems lead to expedited freight and overtime. Since expedited freight and overtime is not included in pricing, we naturally began to experience cash flow shortages. We ended up having to ask customers to find a new supplier for some of the new work in order to regain a proper production flow. I would have been proud of myself that, in 1996, Lewis Metal Stamping booked record sales; however, we also booked record losses on the income statement. That was tough at a tough time, but a lesson well learned.

The transition wasn't without its gender battles. The plant manager, despite his prayer after the news of my father's death, left the company, doubting my capabilities. I fired another plant manager who tried to enter a power struggle with me. I arranged to meet with a man who was struggling in his career at another stamping plant. He came on board and I got to know that he had all the stuff I needed when we had all of the new work. If only I could have had those opportunities once more.

I worked diligently to create my own team and to replace my father's skills. Each time I interviewed prospective staff, I tried to find my father's engineering, quality, and accounting and finance skills. After countless interviews, I realized that I wouldn't find someone to replace my dad. So I hired people with technical skills that I didn't have and relied on myself to understand the finance and accounting as he once instructed me. When I stood back and looked at the operating team, I'd hired all women except for the plant manager. I didn't care because I was comfortable with our team's skill sets and ability to work together as a team. I even had a customer ask if there were any men who worked at the company because his exposure had been only to women. The employee who interfaced with this engineer for new programs was a woman; the accountant who reconciled tool invoices and payment was a woman. I assured him that we keep a man around in case we needed a light bulb changed or something. He laughed.

My new plant manager and I went to an equipment auction to pick up some equipment if it was the right price. At the auction was a man known by all auctioneers and people who went to local manufacturing auctions. This guy owned a used equipment and recycling business that all users of industrial equipment knew about. Mike, my plant manager said, "Whatever you need, you can always find it at this dealer's company."

People attending auctions would moan and grimace when he arrived. They knew that he would outbid anyone if it was something that he really wanted. Although this dealer didn't wear the finest designer suits nor a starched shirt and tie, everyone knew that his pockets were deeper than most.

I knew who he was, but I didn't think he knew who I was. As I checked out a press at the auction he asked, "Aren't you Jim Lewis' wife?" I told him no, I was his daughter. He said, "Oh, wonderful, Jim was a great guy. I really liked him."

He then asked me if I was interested in the press I had been admiring. I told him no—I couldn't afford it at the moment. He said if I was interested that he would not bid on it. I decided we needed it and perhaps I should start replacing some aging equipment. And so I took the plunge. I was bidding against another man and stopped at $40,000. At that time, $40,000 for a press would have been a steal. The other man outbid me at $50,000. When it was all over, I realized that the press was certainly worth more than $50,000 and would have paid for itself in a couple of years. We didn't buy anything but I added the experience to my education. If nothing else it was a learning experience about buying used equipment and the benefit I have of my father's good will.

My next auction was in Ohio. This time my husband and I drove down. I found another press and got into a bidding war with a man from California. He had higher shipping costs to consider than I did. In the middle of our bidding, as I held the highest bid, the auctioneer jeered at the man, "Are you going to let a girl outbid you?" The auctioneer probably made more money with that statement; the other bidder wasn't going to be embarrassed, and at that point, there was no way I was going home without that press. It turned out that the press was perfect for what I needed. It paid for itself in just over two years.

I couldn't believe how excited I was about presses and other support equipment. Some women like furs and diamonds—and I do too. But there was something even more dazzling about a piece of equipment that made money rather than cost money. It was then that I determined that I wasn't just doing this for my dad, I really enjoyed the business. Few women enjoy equipment shopping; most would rather spend

$80,000 on a wardrobe. And don't misunderstand; I like to shop, too. But spending money to make even more money? That's the ticket!

As time passed, I felt more comfortable going out to social business events. People were intrigued with my story—that I was a 31 year-old black female CEO. That intrigue bought me a conversation with some of the movers and shakers in Detroit, and my purpose was to let them know about Lewis Metal Stamping and that it was still in the automotive supply business.

I joined a business association called the National Association of Black Automotive Suppliers. The organization's purpose was to support, educate and promote black automotive suppliers. Each year this group of black auto suppliers awarded four-year scholarships to deserving students going to college to study business or engineering. I gravitated toward the scholarship committee and found myself as one of the presenters at the annual scholarship dinner. At that time there were only two female members and so the administrators managed to always balance the dais with each of us on either side of the speaker among other male NABAS members.

At one of the dinners after the dais was announced and we were waiting for dinner to be served, I noticed a man walking toward me. As he moved into focus I realized that it was my high school friend Richard Chenault. Richard was just as surprised to see me as I was to see him. After quick hellos, he explained that he was attending the dinner as a guest of a friend of his. He told me that he worked for the University of Michigan Transplant Center and wanted to leave some information with me for NABAS to consider supporting the Transplant Center. I of course accepted his materials, and suggested that an organization that my husband belonged to might be an even better fit for him. And that was that. I discussed it with my husband and how the Michigan Funeral Directors might be better poised to support organ donation and transplant, but that was it and I heard no more from Richard.

An Unexpected Mentor

I received an invitation in the mail to an industrial Open House. It was the invitation I had been waiting for from the gentleman I met in Kentucky at Toyota's Minority Supplier Conference. He promised to invite me to his company's Open House. Although they were a stamping supplier to the automotive industry and that would make us competitors, the purpose of the Open House, as the gentleman who I assumed was the CEO explained, was to share ideas, to mix and mingle with customers and collectively find solutions for customer needs. This sounded like a novel idea to me. The idea of an open house designed not solely to showcase the company itself was different and one I hadn't seen before in Detroit. This CEO didn't look like the typical minority supplier in Detroit, nor did his company seem typical. In fact, for someone who represented a minority supplier, he looked to be a white man. Nevertheless, I was interested to model and benchmark something different for Lewis Metal Stamping.

I marked my calendar and since it was in Columbus, Ohio and I had a customer in Columbus, I planned a visit to the customer as well. I visited my customer's plant first and found that the Open House was not far away. When I arrived, there was a buffet area, some standing tables nearby and in another alcove, pictures of the plant, quality charts and blue prints on the wall. Because hors d'oeuvre time was nearly over, I quickly went to the buffet to sample the not-your-average Open House food. Instead of burgers and hotdogs, it was steak skewers with peanut sauce and other gourmet items. I took my plate and browsed through the pictures, parts and charts. I tested myself by reading the blueprints and was pleasantly surprised to find that I could visualize the parts and understand the tolerances, materials, and finishes for the parts. My dad taught me to do that. I pulled my shoulders back and thought, "Maybe I do belong here."

I noticed that there were several employees at the Open House in work uniforms. My 31-year-young naiveté thought "Isn't that nice, he has let the workers in to enjoy some of the food at the Open House." At a table were two of the employees, a black woman and an Asian-Indian man in work uniforms. I went over to the table and said hello and asked in what must have seemed a trite way, "So, what do you do here at the plant?" The woman answered, "I am the Controller", and the gentleman answered, "I am the CFO". I nodded as if I was expecting that answer, and nearly choked on my skewer. Needless to say, what I thought I saw was not what I saw.

Since I had the top brass next to me, I continued my conversation by explaining that I had met the CEO and in fact I was looking for Tony (yeah Tony, that was the guy's name in Kentucky). They looked at me somewhat puzzled. They explained that Francis would be joining us soon. Francis has owned the company for two years now. They were unsure who Tony was. I decided that perhaps I got the name wrong, but surely when the guy Francis comes in, I will recognize him.

Our conversation was interrupted by a stout black man in a work uniform who asked that everyone join him in the alcove where the chairs are set up. I figured to myself that he was opening up for the CEO to take the stage and introduce his customer who will be the guest speaker. I found a seat about half way back and everyone else filled in. As the crowd quieted down, the guy at the podium said, "I am Francis Price. . ." And whatever he said after that, I didn't hear, because it was the last thing I expected him to say. I had to recount everything I had seen thus far that day. I thought to myself, "So do you mean that this magnificent facility in suburban Columbus (and not the lower income section), with a staff that rivals the United Nations in diversity, belongs to a black man?" Francis went on to introduce his customer who likely delivered very eloquent open house remarks. I just don't remember them. All I knew was that I had to know more about this company and this man who owned it. So many of the minority suppliers in Detroit were companies structured as classic 51% minority ownership partnerships or pretenderships. In Detroit, the pretendership seemed to be the only way to capitalize a business. If this company was not one, I had to know so that I could grow Lewis Metal Stamping like that.

After the speaker finished, people broke off into informal discussion groups. I met a few people while I waited for Mr. Price to become available. I introduced myself to him and gave him literature about my small stamping company in Highland Park, MI. He agreed to pass it on to his engineers and was happy that I attended. The social and marketing end of the business has never been my strong suit, so I felt that I had pushed myself and the company quite a bit that day. I was satisfied that it was a day away from the office well spent—a good will visit to a customer and a great learning experience that introduced me to a possible company to model. I jumped into my car and began my four hour drive back to Detroit.

Special Recognition - Black Enterprise Magazine

While sitting in my office opening the mail I received a package express mailed to me. It was from Black Enterprise magazine. The letter had two parts. I had been nominated for an award that would be decided at their annual awards dinner at the culmination of their conference in Orlando, Florida. The second part was that they wanted to do a feature article. Wow! What an honor. How did they know about little old me and my tiny company? In a selfish manner, I thought here's my chance to make up for missing the spread Black Enterprise did on my dad.

A reporter came to the plant and interviewed me. A photographer came later for pictures. The article was published in the August 1996 issue. My next task was to prepare for the awards dinner. Whether I won or lost, it was great to be nominated and even greater to take a vacation in Orlando. I ironically, or as a part of God's divine plan, happened to receive a coupon from an airline company whereby five people could fly for a reduced price. I mentioned it to my mother (knowing she wouldn't miss it for anything in the world) and she told my grandmother, brother and his wife. Seven of us ended up going to the Black Enterprise Magazine Conference for the week. My grandmother, mother, brother, his wife, Steve, Stevie and me, all flew to Orlando. It was fun traveling as one big family.

I attended the conference sessions and of course, we saw lots of Disney. The night of the awards dinner we got dressed early. My hair was short and styled to perfection. My dress was long sleeve, knee length, black and clingy with fading rhinestones from the neckline to the hemline. The dress designer started the dress for a local singer. When the singer decided against the style, I got a beautiful dress, finished to my wishes—fast and reasonably priced. Steve and I left for cocktails and the rest of my family followed on later. We mingled with the important conference participants and corporate sponsors.

Finally the dinner began. The ballroom and tables were decorated as if it were the Academy Awards. It came time to announce the winner of my category. An automotive executive announced the winner, and I could hardly believe that he read my name. Carefully I rose and so did my husband who kissed me, took me by the hand and escorted me to the stage (you know, so I wouldn't fall in those new rhinestone shoes my girlfriend made me buy, and that took both Steve and me to put them on).

I thanked the publisher and awards committee of Black Enterprise magazine and my biggest customer, General Motors. I especially thanked my mother who remained through this struggle the wind beneath my wings. The whole experience seemed so surreal. But I kept in mind what my mentor taught me—don't believe your own propaganda. So I kept it in perspective with all the bad times too.

It was weeks after we went home that my mother showed me a copy of the letter that she wrote the publisher of Black Enterprise magazine months before this award dinner. She congratulated him on his 25th year of being in business and was pleased to see that he chose the November 1991 issue that featured my dad on the cover as the 1991 representative magazine of the 25 years. She went on to tell him that my father had died and that I had taken over the business. My mom then showed me the letter she received back that said "thanks." To this day, I never know how my mom is involved in my work.

❀ ❀ ❀

Chapter Five

The Perfect Plan, or Was It?

A Perfect Plan and a Back-Up Plan

Lewis Metal Stamping was by this time a maturing company of 23 years. In addition to the Black Enterprise magazine recognition, other local media were intrigued by the man-bites-dog story of a young black woman running a manufacturing business. However, although it was novel, the novelty was no benefit to the business and economics of the automotive supply market. Lewis Metal Stamping, despite my best effort, was still growing too slowly and in the grand scheme of things was a tiny supplier to my automotive customers. In order to grow the company quickly enough to survive the '90s climate, I looked for opportunities to merge the company into a larger organization.

My first attempt was one that didn't cause me to fall victim to the popular prescription of minority joint venture ownership, but instead would still allow the entity to be 100% minority owned. The structure would allow me to merge Lewis Metal Stamping into an acquisition that my mentor was making. This business combination opportunity looked strong. It would make us a strong company with viable size.

My mentor allowed me to watch, learn and even participate in this acquisition process. I was able to meet with customers, attorneys, plant personnel and be a part of the entire process as it came together.

We were able to negotiate with customers of the company he was acquiring and get them to agree to not remove their business, but stand still during this process. While they were worried about adding new suppliers to the supply base, we had to convince them that it wouldn't be an addition—just a name change. I met with union officials and was able to assist with constructing a union agreement that would help the combined company be profitable.

After all the due diligence was done, he scheduled closing. The first day was busy with a few last minute clarifications and signatures. On the second day of closing, after insurance was bound and the bank was ready to transfer money, the sellers decided not to sell. What seemed to be a wonderful creation that took the better part of a year to cultivate, didn't happen. The deal that would have been the perfect solution for Lewis Metal Stamping's size disadvantage and the customers needing a viable supplier fell apart. All of the Monday morning quarterbacking and post mortem analysis of the deal suggested that there might have been interference, likely from another supplier, afraid of what our new company might do to the supplier landscape. I shared with my mentor that one way of thinking of this experience is, with all that he had spent on accountants and attorneys for this deal, he had just surpassed my father in education spending for me.

While working on this business combination, I made my major customers aware of the impending changes. Their reaction was positive and they looked forward to our additional capabilities. So when the deal didn't materialize, I needed a plan B—quickly. My second attempt to grow the business, while not as promising from inception, was again an attempt to grow quickly. This time I nearly danced with the devil. I was approached by the operations director of a larger new supplier who recently purchased the assets of a long standing, yet no longer profitable, group of companies. Although they were successful at resizing the business and making the stamping company marginally profitable, they were very profitable at other companies in their automotive technologies portfolio, which made them a profitable group overall. Despite the fact that their interest was in gaining the same benefits that a minority joint venture would provide, they knew that I wouldn't accept those same terms.

What my father always taught me is to know and understand issues myself. He always encouraged me not to rely solely on the advice of professionals but to make sure I understand and agree with what should happen. With that understanding, we formed an agreement whereby I would move onto their campus of stamping operations, rent free. I would have access to their maintenance and engineering staff on a fee-for-service basis. What my collaborators would receive is the benefit of marketing this "Technical Support Agreement" as their efforts to support minority business.

Demise of the Technical Support Agreement

What seemed to be a comfortable way of meeting the objective of growing quickly became difficult. It was no secret that I wanted to buy my technical support partner's stamping operations. This was agreeable from the start with the company's operations director. My mentor helped me to conceptualize how it could be possible. He not only helped me to think about it, but recommended that his CPA firm participate in the process. So the agreement with my technical support agreement partners was that I'd grow Lewis Metal Stamping to a size that would be competitive in the auto industry and purchase their stamping operation to merge with Lewis Metal. Somehow even though there was no exchange of ownership, the relationship still had all the negative connotations of the typical 51-49% minority joint venture.

After I discussed the matter with my CPA, I asked the operations director if I could look at financing the purchase of their stamping operations. He agreed and provided the necessary financial information for us to do a business valuation. What my CPA came up with considering their current book of business, the equipment and real estate, is that the business was worth roughly $10 million dollars. If I were to negotiate a $9 million purchase, it would be a good deal. Understanding that I needed to get Lewis Metal Stamping to a critical mass, I might even be willing to overpay, but not more than $11 million.

I presented this to the Treasurer and Operations Director. They explained that they couldn't do it—not even at the $11 million figure. When they offered no concrete explanation for not being able to do it, I began digging on my own. The company is a publicly traded company and so financial structure and performance information is publicly available.

After reviewing the company's structure, it seems that when my technical support agreement partners purchased the group of companies which included other related technologies, it had to have been the other technologies that were very profitable and compensated for the meager returns brought by the stamping operations. Sure enough, the way that the businesses had been financed, the stamping operations couldn't be separated from their financing agreement, according to public records. It was the assets of the stamping company that was used as collateral for the other businesses which had less equipment to use as collateral. I understood clearly why they couldn't do the deal after understanding how the companies had originally been financed. The other businesses, while technologically superior and sought after by customers, demanded higher prices and yielded higher profits, but took very little equipment. The equipment used for that business was inexpensive. Therefore, when the stamping companies were lumped in with the other businesses, the bank used the capital intensive equipment from the stamping company as collateral and understood that the other businesses would provide income for the whole deal. Therefore, in order to sell the business piece of the package they had to get me to overpay enough to decrease their debt to a level that would satisfy the bank.

I braced myself as customers wanted to award business to Lewis Metal Stamping. It was important to me that the customer wanted their business placed with LMS and not to my technical support partners through me in order to get minority purchasing credit. My TSA (Technical Support Agreement) partners sensed my hesitance and became dismayed with the relationship. I was not doing the job of marketing the association that they wanted to see. In the meantime, they tried to collect revenue by charging for services rendered under the Technical Support Agreement. When maintenance or engineering staff helped us out with a problem, indeed they invoiced us and we paid them. The grey area of the agreement was with the building we occupied and equipment that they left in the building when we moved into their facility. We moved most of our equipment into the building and since the stamping press they left in the building worked, we used it because there was no room to move more of our equipment because of it. The plant manager at the other firm wanted to install hit counters on that press and charge us $.04 per hit.

Our company ran progressive stampings which meant the presses often ran up to 2000 hits per hour. That would mean that we'd pay almost $13,000 per month for use of their press, all the while I had a press at my old plant sitting idle. That certainly didn't make financial sense. There were no other expenses being paid from this press rental. I mean, the price of $04 did not include expenses for utilities or maintenance, I paid for that directly. I explained to my technical support agreement partners that we could abandon the idea of the press hit counters or make the rigging company rich by moving their press out and bringing my press to the building. They agreed to abandon the idea of charging rent for the press.

Finally, we agreed at a meeting that the Technical Support Agreement wasn't bringing the results we expected. However, we didn't agree or even discuss what would be our next steps.

Chapter Six

Perseverance Put to the Test

Kidney Failure

*S*ince my pregnancy, I knew I was spilling significant amounts of protein. My new internist had been working with me over the last year to go on a low protein diet in order to preserve my kidney function. My internist referred me to a nephrologist who saw diabetics from the internist's office.

In January of 2000, after making it through the computer scare of the new millennium at work, my nephrologist explained that I would need to start dialysis. These words fell hard on my ears. All I could think when he said that was that this was the end. From the time I was diagnosed with diabetes and learned about the long term complications of diabetes, I decided that kidney failure was the complication I would most want to avoid. I figured I could live and be blind or without a limb, but I couldn't live without kidney function.

I left the doctor's office still contemplating what dialysis would mean to my life, my family and my business. I returned to the office. The mail was in and I began to triage it. I always triaged mail for the important stuff—stuff time sensitive or critical to the business, leaving all the other mail for the secretary to distribute later. In the mail was a letter from the court system. Inside was an eviction notice from my partners in the Technical Support Agreement. Evidently they decided what the next course of action should be; they just didn't have the intestinal fortitude to discuss it face to face with me. I found out their wishes via registered mail in the form of an eviction notice.

Meanwhile my nephrologist explained the difference between peritoneal dialysis and hemodialysis. In hemodialysis patients go to a dialysis clinic three times a week and connect to a machine while literally all of the patient's blood is pumped out, cleaned and pumped back in. A shunt is surgically inserted into the vein for easier and more secure connection to the dialysis machine. This process is invasive and makes the patient very tired for several hours afterwards. My doctor, while he explained the process, never really saw this as a viable option for me. The other type of dialysis is peritoneal dialysis, which is done with a surgically inserted catheter and uses the peritoneum (the sack that holds your organs together) as a filter to clean the blood. Two liters of dialysis fluid remains in the peritoneum until the next exchange scheduled every other hour. The patient then connects the drainage bag to the catheter and empties the old fluid, and fills the abdomen with new fluid. The fluid surrounds veins and capillaries in the abdomen pulling out waste deposited into the bloodstream. It also removes excess fluid from the body that the kidneys no longer remove. New fluid is added to the abdomen using an IV pole and gravity. The whole process takes about a half hour and repeats every other hour, unless a machine called a cycler is used during the night. The way a cycler works is in the evening the patient connects him or herself to the cycler machine using hoses and a drainage tube that reaches and empties into to the toilet, and one that connects to ten liters of fresh fluid warming on top of the cycler. The reason that it is called a cycler is because one cycle consists of one drain and fill cycle. Ideally, the overnight dialysis consists of moving ten liters of fluid through the body. The fluid is held in the abdomen in order to pull the impurities out of the bloodstream, ideally for an hour. The number of cycles that are actually completed depends on the time set for completion on the cycler. Therefore if I was late getting connected or had an early morning meeting and had to disconnect early, then I missed a few cycles and wasn't able to make full use of the cycler. The ideal setting was to maximize the hold-time at two hours and complete five cycles, moving ten liters of fluid during the night. The total connection time was approximately 8 hours. Given my busy schedule both at work and at home, my nephrologist gave me the choice, but strongly recommended peritoneal dialysis with a cycler.

I anticipated needing to be up getting my son ready for school, and that meant I had to disconnect from the cycler by

6:30 a.m. Therefore I needed to get connected no later than 9 p.m. I made sure the tubing was long enough to get to the bathroom and, later, to the computer since 9 p.m. was after homework was generally completed and I could finish my own work.

When my nephrologist decided that I needed to start dialysis, they were the words I should have been anticipating and should have been prepared to hear for a long time, but they weren't. I scheduled lunch with my husband, mother and brother. I know that sounds so formal but this was an issue that required a serious, away from the distractions of home, discussion. I didn't want my son within ear shot until I knew exactly what I would do and how to best present it to him. After we ordered our meal, I told them that my kidneys had failed and that I was going to start dialysis. Before I could get it all out, I broke down into tears. I quickly recovered; after all we were in public. I explained to them that I would have surgery to have a catheter inserted, and how the dialysis process would work. I also explained how tired the kidney failure was making me and that I doubted whether I would be able to continue to run the business. My brother has been used to a hard-working sister, in school and at work, who had never given up. To hear this was foreign to his ears. He innocently asked, "So what will you do then?" I told him I would somehow get a job.

Since I wasn't sure how this might turn out in the long run, I asked them not to tell anyone. Of course my son would know because he lived in the house, and I would explain it to him correctly. My mother asked if she could tell my grandmother and I agreed as long as she didn't tell anyone else.

So our little secret began. A little secret became a huge cover up. The most important reason for not wanting people to be aware of my kidney failure is because of the business implications. I didn't want employees, customers, suppliers and other business associates to know because my illness could become a threat to the success or existence of Lewis Metal Stamping. It could blow out of proportion in the automotive business community, as many things do. However, my immediate and first reason for not wanting anyone to know about my kidney failure is because it was simply bad news. It was bad news that I didn't have a solution for. I never want to present a problem without a solution and for this I didn't have even a potential solution. It hurt me to have to tell immediate family that I had to start dialysis. So I chose not to tell others. My immediate family was a part of my everyday life and I had to not only let them know what was going on, but I had to also depend on them.

Understanding all of the new requirements of dialysis also meant that going on vacation would be difficult, and field trips at my son's school would be out of the question—especially the overnight 3rd grade Nature Camp field trip. So I asked my nephrologist if I could postpone dialysis until after nature camp. That would allow me not only to spend some quality time with my son as a normal mom, but also complete some other important things that month.. And so my nephrologist agreed to postpone dialysis.

Third grade culminated in a four day field trip to Nature Camp. My nephrologist was trying to schedule me to have surgery to begin dialysis. This wasn't emergency surgery and so I asked him to allow me to complete three events that were very important to me. The first was to be a chaperone when my son went to Nature Camp, attend a spa trip with girlfriend colleagues in Palm Springs and satisfy a commitment to present scholarships at the annual NABAS fund-raising dinner. All of it would be complete in 30 days and he obliged me as long as I understood warning signs requiring me to go to a hospital emergency room immediately. If I felt heart palpitations or shortness of breath, my diastolic blood pressure was likely more than 100, and I should go immediately to the emergency room.

I was so happy that he understood my need to go on this field trip. I certainly couldn't do this while on dialysis. And who knew how long I would even enjoy being here on earth with my son. The trip to Palm Springs was important, too, because I had already completely paid for it and it turned out to be an incredible trip that my girlfriends and I will remember for the rest of our lives. It was a rare sort of professional female bonding and spiritual uplifting for women of color. The three of us were in need of that uplifting experience for our own individual reasons. And the NABAS scholarship dinner was something uplifting and an event that I was committed to complete. I am so glad that my nephrologist allowed me these important interruptions to my start of dialysis.

I didn't take these trips without calculating the risks and what I would do in a worse case situation. Another girlfriend, also a parent at the school, was coming to chaperone the trip. Although she didn't know that I was scheduled to begin dialysis soon, I knew that if I were in need of emergency attention, she is a physician and would make sure I got the attention that I needed. It would mean that I would have to come clean with my secret of kidney failure, but it was a secret I was willing to break if medically necessary.

The nature camp experience was one that every parent should have. Being in the outdoors, watching my son study science in nature as well as share other outdoor activities with his classmates was fun. To see him hold KP responsibilities gave me good ideas for home. Kidney failure and the resulting anemia, made me weak and not able to recover from a misstep easily, and sometimes not at all. A couple times while walking up the hill from the girls' cabin to the mess hall I tripped on a stone on the dirt road and skinned my knee. I managed to do it twice in one day on the same knee. It wasn't a horrific fall, just a simple stumble. But because I wasn't able to react quickly enough and catch my fall or brace myself, the fall caused my knee to bleed. I didn't have a band aid and didn't want to draw attention to myself by asking for one, so I sat at the camp fire with my hand over my knee where the blood soaked through my jeans.

My trip to the spa in Palm Springs was more than a relaxing visit to the spa. It was a spirit-filled time for me and two girlfriends. Despite my nosebleed from high blood pressure (caused by the kidney failure) the whole flight from Detroit to LA, I don't think I've laughed more in my life! For instance, the trip began with my change in travel itincrary.

One girlfriend booked us on first class travel from Detroit to Palm Springs. We call that girlfriend, The Queen. I saved us half the fare by booking a red-eye from Detroit to Los Angeles, and then taking a taxi from L.A. to Palm Springs. What I forgot about was the fatigue from the four hour flight from Detroit to L.A. and I didn't anticipate another three hour cab ride from L.A. to Palm Springs. Let me sum it up by saying that we arrived at the Palm Springs resort at 2 a.m. Each of us grabbed our keys from the desk clerk and without saying anything to the other and went to our respective rooms.

Another hilarious moment was after the hair and make-up sessions, the three of us went shopping for beauty items to preserve our look—at the 24-hour drug store of course. My girlfriend Jackie wanted to buy some rollers to preserve the curly look she received at the salon. Earlier she purchased $400 worth of makeup brushes during the makeup session. As we searched through the convenience drug store for rollers, Jackie was appalled by the seemingly high price of $4 for the pack of rollers. Now remember, she had just left the posh surroundings of our Palm Springs resort and spent $400 on makeup brushes. I had to remind her that perhaps if she had only spent $396 on the makeup brushes, then $4 for the rollers wouldn't seem so bad. The camaraderie, pampering, and spiritual closeness with my girlfriends were more than I could have ever hoped for.

In the middle of May 2000, I finally had outpatient surgery for the catheter for peritoneal dialysis. Dialysis centers and dialysis wards in the hospital always have older people in them and the center or unit smells like urine. So I dreaded this whole experience. In the area where they prepped me, there was a guy about my age who was getting his second catheter. The first was removed because he got peritonitis (an infection of the peritoneum). He did hemodialysis until the infection was cleared. The nurse at the dialysis clinic said to always monitor my drainage fluid to make sure it was clear and not cloudy. Cloudy fluid is a symptom of peritonitis.

Somehow I felt better that there was someone my age going through the same thing. My surgery was on a Friday and I recuperated over the weekend. The following Monday morning I reported to the dialysis clinic to begin my week long training. The training was supposed to take two weeks and the doctor knew that I couldn't take that much time away, so he and the nurse designed an abbreviated one-week version that would include the advanced training on hooking up to the cycler (overnight dialysis machine) overnight.

My first dialysis treatment was scheduled for the Monday after surgery at the dialysis center. I spent the weekend healing from surgery. On Monday morning I met my nurse, Pam. She gave me a surgical mask to wear and masked herself. Pam gently unwrapped my gauze and cleaned the area with an antiseptic wipe. She explained that she would perform the dialysis today and that we would do them together Tuesday through Thursday and on Friday she would watch me do it. After that, I would be on my own. So carefully she started with half a liter of fluid and after two hours of holding the fluid, she showed me how it drew excess fluid off of my body by draining a whole liter. After lunch we tried a full liter. Again after two hours, we drained almost two liters. The dialysis was taking the stored fluid off of my body—off of my ankles, away from my heart and lungs, out of my swollen tissue all over my body. More importantly it was removing the waste from my blood stream that my kidneys were unable to get rid of. She explained the purpose of ramping up to the standard 2 liter fluid amount was to slowly stretch my peritoneum to do what we needed it to do.

We went through the process enough times that she felt comfortable enough to let me try at home. On Thursday of that week, she showed me how to set up my cycler machine and I received my very own machine to take home. She gathered all of my supplies and explained how the fluid company would deliver once per month and that I should keep good inventory of each of the fluid strengths. Dialysis fluid comes in three strengths: 1.5, 2.5 and 4.0. The higher the fluid number, the stronger the dialysis fluid and the more fluid it would remove from my body. I came to differentiate them as 1.5 for when my blood pressure was normal and any other strength would lower my blood pressure to the point of being dizzy. Fluid strength 2.5 is the moderate fluid strength. While stronger than 1.5, it pulled more fluid and was effective when my blood pressure was moderately high. The 4.0 fluid, or the "theatre popcorn" fluid as I called it, cured all sins—theatre popcorn, pizza, the sodium works. During the training session Pam described different things that might occur so that I wouldn't become frightened. For instance she explained that because the ovaries and fallopian tubes are not connected, the fluid sometimes can get into and drain out of the uterus. In that case, the drainage fluid may be slightly pink. But under no circumstances should I see bright red blood. If I did, I should go to the ER immediately. Well, just as she predicted one night I noticed that the drainage fluid in the tube was pink and I became afraid. I woke my husband up and we called the dialysis nurse on call. She asked a few questions including if I was of child bearing years, and calmly explained that it was likely blood from my uterus. I should add 1 cc of heparin to my dialysis bag to make sure I didn't clot.

The nurses at the dialysis center were dialysis experts and compassionate souls. I came to the dialysis center so afraid of what would happen. In fact, I thought I would die. All the nurses, but Pam in particular, calmed my fears.

With the number of friends and family that my husband and I have, it was near impossible to keep this news from everyone. My dear friend and colleague, Jackie, stopped by my house because I missed a meeting for the NABAS Scholarship. I explained my reason was because I had to have some minor surgery. Concerned, she decided rather than ask the question and pry, she would drop by my house to check on me after my surgery. Well I am not a good liar, and besides she was the only other woman member of this business association we belonged to, so perhaps I could confide in her. After hearing the news, she sighed, asked if there was anything she could do, and made sure that I understood that if there was anything that I needed, I could call on her. I was sure that she would hold my confidence and more importantly, hold me up in prayer.

My secret was again uncovered when my college roommate, Thea, was in the area and dropped by my house with her mother. Well, as they arrived, my son was leaving the house to ride his bike. They knocked at the door, several times. They asked Stevie where I was and why hadn't I opened the door? Stevie told them, "Oh, wait a minute, she'll be down. She is doing an exchange." When I finally answered the door, quite naturally, Thea asked, "What is an exchange?" So I had to explain.

Although I was not dishonest with my condition when confronted directly, I didn't want to watch the sorrow on people's face when I said the words, "I am in kidney failure and I am on dialysis." There were some people that I specifically didn't want to know about my kidney failure. Friends who worked in the medical profession who watch people die of kidney failure all the time, would be especially hurt. I knew that I wouldn't be able to fight if I was constantly looking into the sorrow filled faces of friends and family. So I tried to maintain the secret.

At home, I got to be a real pro at dialysis and monitoring my health. Each night before bed, my husband would lug ten liters of dialysis fluid from a storage room upstairs to our bedroom so that I could connect to my cycler. While my husband complained about most chores, he never complained about carrying nearly 20 pounds of fluid to our bedroom each night in order to sustain my life. My diabetes regimen was now an even more complicated set of processes. Each day after disconnecting from the dialysis cycler, I would test my blood sugar, blood pressure, weigh myself (to check for excessive fluid weight gain or loss), record all the results for the doctor to review at my visits, take my insulin and eat according to the rules of not only diabetes but of dialysis. My body couldn't clear phosphorus from my system, so I had to take a pill before any type of meal. This agent would bind to phosphorus in my system so that it could be excreted in my stool. I also had to watch the amount of potassium I ate. Potatoes were cut from my diet unless I soaked them overnight, drained the water, and rinsed them again before cooking them. Citrus fruit was out as well as tomatoes or foods made with tomato sauce, because of the high potassium in them. Watching my blood pressure and blood sugar was key to remaining healthy while on dialysis. My dialysis nurse explained that I should use different strengths of fluid depending on how much water I needed to take off my body.

Once I had the dialysis procedure memorized I could then start to fit this extra monitoring more smoothly into my daily schedule. I had to hold each type of fluid in my monthly inventory of fluid at work as well as at home. I didn't let kidney failure run my life. I incorporated dialysis into my daily routine.

Once I had a meeting at 1 p.m. and a busy day scheduled. I worked right up until 12:15 and had a ½ hour drive to make. I had postponed dialysis in the past and felt sluggish, so I decided not to try it again. I packed up my dialysis supplies into a spare briefcase and took it to my car. I slipped the mask on in the parking lot and carefully and cleanly connected. I put the drainage bag on the passenger side floor and the new bag on my dash to heat up in the sun while I drove to the meeting and drained the old dialysis fluid out. When I finished draining, I switched the dam on the bags so that the new fluid could enter. Although the dash was above my heart, gravity allowed the fluid to fill my peritoneal cavity, but pinching the bag in the sunroof of my car worked even better. At a red light, I again washed my hands with the antibacterial wipe and put the mask back over my face and disconnected from the bags. I taped and secured my hose and clamped the old fluid and put it back into the bag and into the trunk of my car. I attended the meeting as planned and felt good during and after it.

I had monthly visits with the dialysis team. They drew my blood first and the dietician monitored many of my blood values including my creatinine. Creatinine is a measure of kidney function. Normal creatinine is below 2.0. My creatinine was 9 but dialysis had brought it to 7.

Because I had become so tired and not very productive before dialysis, I noticed that instead of my normal 5:30 a.m. wake-up I didn't get to work until 9:30 or 10 a.m. Keeping up with my son's activities was a challenge despite iron vitamins. Dialysis chewed up my red blood cells which caused my iron to be low. The fix for low hemoglobin (anemia) was a weekly injection of a drug called Epotin which increased my energy level.

As a result of the eviction from my TSA partners, my operating team and I had to plan to relocate the business. While we looked at other buildings available in the area, nothing made better sense than to move back into our buildings in Highland Park. Moving industrial equipment is no easy or inexpensive task. Fortunately we turned negative cash flow into positive cash flow and built some reserves. In order to move back into the buildings, we had to refurbish and renovate the buildings. We had to notify our customer base as well as build banks of parts to ship while our equipment was being moved and reinstalled.

The rigging company moved the equipment first and we scheduled office movers to move the office equipment and the computer technicians moved and reinstalled the computer equipment. Tired from the strain of dialysis, I didn't arrive at the office the morning of the office move until almost 9 a.m. The movers had already arrived and the staff was directing them. As I walked up to the building, one of the movers was requesting payment before he got started. My controller (a white woman) explained that paying in advance wasn't how we operated, that we would pay upon completion. Other staff members stopped to listen to this strange request. When I came into the office, my controller explained the situation to me. When I asked the mover what the problem was, he explained that he was concerned about getting paid, especially since the company was moving from Clinton Township (a white northeastern suburb of Detroit) to Highland Park (a black city that is an island inside of Detroit). After a racist comment like that I decided that this was not a company that we wanted to pay at all, nor did we want to entrust our belongings with them. I explained that we would find another mover and asked him to return the items he had loaded onto his truck. He then informed me that I would need to pay the $300 minimum call fee and do so in cash.

The Clinton Township police was located just down the street and I asked my controller to call them to handle this dispute. The officer came to our plant and read the fine print on the contract (signed by my production control manager) which obligated us to the $300 call fee payable in cash. The police officer agreed with me that this was a racist scum bag company, however he couldn't do anything about the obligation.

Our business is not a cash business, and our petty cash rarely exceeded $300. Fortunately we had the cash. My controller gave me the $300 and as I walked out to pay the scum bag and made sure the police witnessed their return of our property, my Engineering Manager walked up from the parking lot. He had $300 in his hand and wanted to give it to me to pay the movers. Disgusted by what he had witnessed, he told me that he went to his ATM to get the cash. Somehow this mover's racist behavior didn't seem as bad anymore. After taking care of the mover and being assured that our property would be returned, I realized that through this incident, my white Engineering Manager had a chance to see what racism felt like first hand. This mover's racist views and actions had affected my engineering manager's ability to help get us out of this situation. The fact that he would offer to use his own money to side step this obstacle said more about this man than the engineering function he performed.

Qualifying For Kidney Transplant

I knew that dialysis couldn't last forever. Unless I got a kidney transplant, I would die. However, the transplant process is not simply find one and get it transplanted. The waiting list for cadaveric kidneys averages 5 years. I didn't know if I could make it that long, but fortunately for me, my brother didn't give me enough time to wonder whether I could. Not long after my dialysis started, he said that he would give me one of his kidneys. He said it with such confidence that we never considered what if he wasn't a match. So Jeff and I underwent the antigen matching process. We were pretty sure that we'd match since we had the same blood type. For his role in my pregnancy, Jeff banked blood for my C-section.

Indeed we matched 4 of 6 antigens; 3 is considered a good match and they sometimes transplant others with fewer matching antigens. So Jeff was a match and healthy enough to donate, however, I had to undergo extensive medical and psychological testing to qualify as a transplant recipient. Just as I was about to undergo testing and be officially placed on the organ transplant list at a local community hospital, I thought it was a good idea to call my friend Richard who was a member of the transplant team at the University of Michigan hospital; Richard was my high school friend who brought "water" to the girls softball team, and who I ran into at the NABAS scholarship banquet. I decided that it would be a good idea to just talk to him about the transplant process and what to expect, even though I was at another hospital.

When I talked to Richard, he was surprised and saddened to hear that I was on dialysis and needed a kidney transplant. He explained the transplant list process and how the surgery is typically performed. He then explained in a politically correct manner the differences in surgical practices and organ selection among hospitals. I hung up the phone and as I began considering what he said, I thought to myself, "Why would I go anywhere other than my alma mater? Not just my alma mater, but one of the top transplant programs in the country." So even though Jeff and I were typed and matched at our local community hospital, we agreed that we wanted the transplant performed at the University of Michigan Transplant Center.

At our first appointment, the doctors repeated the antigen match test. I then had to go through a battery of tests in order to qualify for a transplant. I was evaluated by a social worker who not only considered my state of mind and family support situation, but they also evaluated my insurance and ability to not only pay for the transplant, but for post transplant medication that I would need to take for the rest of my life. The post transplant medication without insurance costs about $17,000 per year. For some, not being able to afford the medication without insurance is the reason for transplant rejection. Therefore in order to be a good candidate for a kidney transplant, not only do you need the ability to pay for the transplant, but also for the life sustaining drugs for the rest of your life.

I was interviewed by several medical professionals who not only evaluated my medical ability to withstand transplant surgery, but also assessed whether I was a compliant patient— in other words, they wanted to know if I would follow the regimen as prescribed in order to protect my new kidney or would I fall into habits that would jeopardize my new kidney, like drinking alcohol excessively, smoking or not taking my medication. The physical tests included an EKG, cardiac stress test, chest X-ray, and regular gynecological tests as well as clearance from my dentist who made sure I had all dental work complete and no decay in my mouth. With green lights in all the categories, I was cleared for surgery.

It was Jeff who called to schedule surgery. I had gone through all of this because it was also necessary for me to be listed for a cadaveric kidney on the transplant list. I had to be listed even if I had my own living related donor. But in my mind I wasn't sure that I wanted my brother to go through this. I desperately wanted to see my son grow up, but I didn't want to put my brother in any danger. Jeff called me at work to tell me the date: December 14, 2000. It was a good date for him because he was done with school finals, and he figured it would be a good date for me because the auto companies were shut down the last two weeks in December for the holidays. It was a good date, and I didn't have time to ponder, what if.

So I began to make plans to be away from the office a few days before the holiday shut-down. All through dialysis I kept my illness a secret, especially from employees. So about two weeks before my surgery, I told my operating team. I explained to them that I was on dialysis and would receive my brother's kidney. It felt ok, telling people that I was on dialysis this way, because I had a transplant solution. To just say that I was on dialysis sounded fatal. I told my administrative assistant that I planned to return for the Christmas Party, if only for a little while.

Our Kidney Transplant

Jeff and I went to the hospital to have final pre-surgery exams a week before the transplant date. For the most part we were in the exam room together so that the physician's assistant could get a family history and a basic listen to our hearts and lungs. Jeff had a slight cough, but the doctor said it wasn't enough to cancel surgery. Then they separated us. I thought it was to do a more extensive exam, but it was to give Jeff one final chance to change his mind. The doctor asked him if he was under any pressure to do the surgery and if he would like to back out. If so, he just became too sick to have surgery. Jeff said no, he was ready to go. The doctor gave me prescriptions for two of the anti-rejection medications that I would be taking. He wanted me to start the medicine two days before the transplant. My instructions were to connect to my cycler the night before, and with the last cycle, not refill my abdomen with fluid. As the doctor said, "Come in dry."

The transplant was scheduled for December 14, 2000, a Tuesday morning, at 7 a.m. I had Monday to complete and tie things up at work and at home. I arranged for my mother to sign payroll checks and to be available to sign checks for any emergency financial matter. I left instructions for all the staff and had full confidence that they could handle things while I was gone. That Monday it snowed terribly. There was 6+ inches of snow on the ground for my evening commute home.

My car got stuck in the snow in my driveway when I tried to pull up. I left it right where it got stuck for my husband to deal with because I had a long list of things around the house to do before I did my last dialysis cycle. In order for it to be a complete 10 cycles before I had to disconnect at 5 a.m. and leave for Ann Arbor the next morning, I needed to be connected by 7 or 7:30 p.m. Arriving home at 6: 30 p.m. meant I had only an hour or an hour and a half to get my running around done.

Earlier in the week, I washed and ironed my son's school uniforms and prepared the house for me to be gone for a while. What I didn't think to do and wish I did was pack an overnight bag for myself. I was so focused on the transplant itself, I didn't even think to pre pack my own toothpaste, hair brush, etc.

I got connected to my dialysis cycler late. In fact it was 11 p.m. before I was sure the house was prepared to be without me. When I programmed the cycler with a completion time, it adjusts the fluid hold time in order to go through ten cycles. It turned out that I had to cut back to less than 30 minutes hold time, as opposed to the normal hour for my last dialysis session. Nevertheless, I connected.

The next morning I disconnected from the cycler and manually drained all of the fluid from my abdomen. I've had surgeries before and I know that if my blood sugar is out of control, then they may cancel surgery. I couldn't afford for this to happen since this was the ideal time for both Jeff and I to have surgery. And if for any reason they decided not to do the surgery, the disappointment would be unbearable. So I tested my blood sugar to make sure it was within an acceptable range. When I tested it was nearly 400. Normal range is 70-120, and they would likely still continue up to about 200, but 400 was not acceptable. Doctors cancelled my mother's back surgery because her blood sugar was too high. There was so much anticipation for this day, and the time worked out perfect for Jeff and me. So, although I was instructed not to take any insulin or eat any food, I needed to bring this blood sugar down. I took 4 units of Humalog. Humalog is a fast-acting, short-lasting insulin that would get into my system to bring the blood sugar down in 15 minutes, yet it wouldn't still be working for 12 or 24 hours. It would be completely out of my system in 8 hours. The anesthesiologist manages my glucose levels during surgery by administering insulin or glucose intravenously. I was only interested in getting a starting blood sugar that was reasonable. I knew it would be managed during surgery. I don't recommend that anyone try this at home. It was a very calculated noncompliance on my part.

I forgot how slim I could look without carrying the two liters of fluid in my belly. As I got dressed I was able to get into my skinny jeans without cutting off blood circulation to my legs. Adequate blood flow in my groin area was critical since that is where they intended to put Jeff's kidney.

On December 14, 2000 Jeff met us at 6:00 a.m. at my house in the big snow storm. I had a last minute LMS deposit to make so Jeff went ahead to meet Mom to caravan to U of M Hospital. Steve and Stevie and I met them in Ann Arbor. The surgical waiting room seemed busy for so early in the morning. Soon they called Jeff and me back to prepare. Jeff got undressed and into his hospital gown while they tested my potassium to make sure we could proceed with surgery. My potassium level was perfect. And so they put Jeff's IV in and gave him the surgical uniform—cute little socks and a bonnet to match. The nurse made a last call of relatives to come see Jeff before surgery so I went to get his wife, son, Mom, Steve, Stevie and Jeff's mother-in-law. We all kissed him and said, "See you in recovery."

All of a sudden this was real. It was really going to happen. Jeff was going to give me his left kidney. Up until this point I had been so strong; so matter of fact about this whole ordeal. But to see Jeff in the hospital gown about to undergo major surgery--for me, was overwhelming. I grabbed his hand and told him how overwhelmed I was and that I loved him so much. A little woozy from the "feel good" the anesthesiologist gave him, he said. "I love you too, big sis." And they wheeled him away.

Jeff later told me that when he went into the operating room, he could see the surgeons scrubbing while the nurses were prepping him for surgery. He asked if they would get the surgeon for him. When they asked why, he told them because he wanted to see the surgeon's eyes and shake his hand. They got the surgeon and he leaned down and looked into Jeff's eyes. He shook Jeff's hand and told him that he would take good care of him. Jeff said, "Thanks." And that's all he remembers.

This was all at about 8:00 a.m. Meanwhile in the surgical waiting room, my son and Jeff's son and mother-in-law played Monopoly. Jeff's wife later took the kids to eat breakfast. Mom's best friend came to be with her while both of mom's kids were in surgery. Steve read all of the magazines in the surgical waiting area. My sister-in-law and her mother again took the kids to eat lunch. My girlfriend's daughter, in school at the University of Michigan at the time, came bearing a gift of apples with a scripture written on the bag. And me, I sat there starving since I hadn't had anything to eat since midnight the night before. My friend Richard said that the surgeons took longer than expected because Jeff had so much muscle mass to cut and everyone in the operating room was remarking about how BIG the kidney was. A Perfusionist colleague scrubbed in on the surgery, charged with monitoring the kidney between surgeries, called Richard back and said, "Dude, check out the size of this kidney!"

It was my turn. I got dressed as I had so many times before—my eye surgery, my C-section, my laparoscopy, my catheter for dialysis. My abdomen looks like an NFL playbook. I know the routine. IV, a little oral indigestion medicine and then a hit in the IV of "feel good". The next trick for me is to try to remember the last thing I saw before lights out. Mom, her girlfriend, Steve, Stevie and I had prayer. Steve gave me a kiss. And that's all I remember!

It was now after 11 p.m. It had been a long day for our family. I'm told that when the surgeons came out to say that the kidney was functioning and they were sewing me up, my 9-year-old son had a question for the surgeon. Please understand that Stevie had some concern before the surgery that only specialists would work on his uncle and mom. I assured him then that surgeons and nephrologists would be our doctors. And so when the surgeon came out to give the family an update, Stevie asked if they were still sewing his mom up, why then was he (the surgeon) out there talking to the family? My husband explained the roles and responsibilities of surgeons and surgical residents to Stevie. After understanding the required education to become a surgical resident, he felt much better.

Although it was so late, the doctors allowed Stevie to visit and hold hands with me in recovery. Mom, Stevie, Steve and our pastor visited for a few short minutes and assured me that Jeff was doing fine. The family had to leave so that the doctors could put a central line in my neck. I remember the resident telling another resident that he had been instructed to start the central line and that his supervisor would be there shortly to complete it. I listened as he had some concern that he was doing this alone and would prefer some supervision. Thank God for anesthesia drugs, otherwise I too might have been concerned. As he finished, he said, "I did it. I'm the man!" He thought I was asleep. I said, "Yeah, you the man! You the man!" He said, "What, you heard me?" I smiled. Every time this resident came by for rounds, he could never look me in the eye. I pretended not to remember the incident.

Friday morning Jeff and I found that we were directly across the hall from one another. That made it easy for our family to visit both of us. My surgical team went to visit Jeff, explaining that they wanted to shake the hand of the guy who donated the biggest kidney they had ever transplanted. This really must be some kidney!

The doctors grew concerned as my urine output dropped from 300 cc to 75 cc. They sent me down for an ultrasound to find that my blood flow to Jeff's huge kidney was just fine. Chuck, the physician's assistant who is self described as a "cowboy from Wyoming," explained to me that Jeff usually has a beer to jump start his kidney, so that's what he'll probably have to prescribe for me. My nephrologist prescribed more water and indeed my urine output increased.

Concerned about reports that my new kidney may be experiencing some rejection, Jeff ventured out with Foley bag and IV in toe, across the hall to visit. There was no better sight to my eyes than to see my baby brother in his mini dress hospital gown pushing his IV with a pee bag hanging on the side. He later told me he had a rookie nurse helping him out of bed. She took off running with the Foley catheter. He had to explain to her that neither he nor the lead was that long and she should wait for him to catch up with her.

Each day brought us more strength and fewer pushes on the pain IV or as Jeff called it, "dope on a rope." Soon I was able to visit across the hall in Jeff's room. I met his roommate who received a cadaveric kidney the day after our surgery. He was on his way out of town on a business trip when he received a page from the hospital. He didn't board the plane and instead went to the hospital to change his life forever.

By Tuesday, we packed our bags and headed home. It is still amazing to imagine that in five days we had surgery and were well enough to go home—and we were happy to go home. It was great to tell the lunch tray person, "no thanks—no gruel for me—I'm goin' home!" Steve and my sister-in-law picked us up and we went home together.

Mom took us both for our one-week check up. It was like being kids again. She held our coats while they drew our blood. She was in the zone—she had her babies back again. The doctors said Jeff was healing well and was released from transplant care. His regular doctor now monitors him. My follow-up visits would continue weekly until my blood values were at clinical levels and my medication doses were stable.

At home, Mom served as our prison warden, making us eat all the right foods and making sure we got rest. When she went to check on Jeff's cell block, she left The Enforcer, Granny, in charge at my house. Granny made me take a nap at 3:00 in the afternoon like I was 4 years old. And I went to sleep too. The most noticeable difference in having a functioning kidney was my energy level. I felt like I could conquer the world. Prednisone gave me a pretty good boost, too, but putting out that golden ale called urine—it's an amazing thing.

The radio station Jeff worked for called him at home to do an interview about the transplant. During a follow up interview, the DJ told Jeff on the air that his interview right after the surgery touched a 13-year-old girl who was at the mall from which they were broadcasting. She had been through three kidney transplants and she thought it was wonderful that Jeff had donated a kidney to his sister.

Post-Kidney Transplant Management—
Replacing One Disease Regimen with Another

During my pre-transplant screening, doctors were careful to describe my transplant as "treatment" for my kidney failure. It was not a cure because in the beginning, there is as much as a 20% chance of me rejecting the transplanted kidney. In fact they said that acute rejection was likely within the first five years of transplant and that I should plan on it. And so I started the rest of my life with a new regimen of immunosuppression and a different set of metrics to monitor.

Two months after my kidney transplant the surgeon scheduled removal of my Tenkoff Catheter. This was the surgically implanted hose that I used for dialysis. The protocol is to wait two months to make sure the kidney is functioning. They don't wait much longer because it can be a source of infection. And infection is a transplant patient's worst nightmare. The catheter was removed as outpatient surgery and was relatively uneventful.

Later that month, after dinner one day, I developed a terrible stomachache. The pain was so tremendous I called my husband home from a board meeting. We went to the hospital that put in and removed my catheter for them to evaluate me. I was unable to hold anything down—not even water. Doctors tried to get me to drink contrast in order to do an MRI; however I would throw up the contrast before they could get the test started.

The doctors wanted to get everything off of my stomach to alleviate the production of gas and swelling in my stomach. So they inserted an NG tube through my nose to my stomach to suction off any food or liquid that was there causing gas to build up. Never, never, as long as you live, let anyone insert an NG tube while you are conscious! You need to be completely relaxed for the procedure, and I'm sorry, it is impossible to relax while someone pushes a tube up your nose and down your esophagus. The nurse came in to explain its purpose and how she would insert the tube. She had a cup of water and when she said "swallow," I was to swallow while she inserted the tube. I gagged after a few attempts. Soon others came to help her. It seems the difficulty was with her stuttering. When she said sa-sa-swallow, I didn't know on which "sa" I should begin swallowing. The tube was eventually inserted, but not without scratching the back of my throat. After surgery, Steve asked his friend, an ear, nose and throat doctor, to evaluate the damage. His colleague came to see me and said that indeed it was irritated, but in time it would heal.

After nearly 24 hours on Dilauded for pain, the doctors surmised that it must be a hernia. However there was no way to know for sure because I was unable to complete the MRI. So they scheduled exploratory surgery and if indeed it was a hernia, they would make the necessary repairs at the same time.

My intense pain caused doctors to move relatively quickly. This happened on a Wednesday night and Thursday was payroll transfer day. When the doctors decided that it was time to go to surgery, I paged my husband and called my mother. Shortly after my page, my husband happened to be on his way to the hospital so he came on up to the room instead of calling first. He listened as the surgical resident explained the procedure and what they expected to find. I talked with my mother and explained that they were going to do surgery.

She of course wanted to come to the hospital to see me, but I explained that Steve was with me and that I needed her to pick up my son from school when he got out at 3 p.m. I explained that I also needed her to sign payroll checks today and there were two other checks from the general account that needed to go out this week, too. We exchanged I love yous and hung up.

I then called the office to explain where I was and what was about to happen. I spoke with the controller to get the payroll liability—the amount of money needed in the payroll account to cover the payroll checks, electronic transfers, and payroll taxes. I told her to expect my mother to come in to sign the payroll checks and that I would transfer the funds prior to surgery. My controller was new and didn't yet have bank transfer privileges. In the midst of my dialing the bank, the resident waiting to take me to the operating room became impatient with my preparations and said, "I can't believe this!" I paused my dialing and asked him to get over himself. I told him, "There's much more to life than just you and I." I called the automated phone service and transferred the payroll liability from the general account to the payroll account and noted the confirmation number. I asked my husband to make sure the controller got the confirmation number for her records.

My surgeon was completing a surgery in another operating room when they wheeled me down. The operating room schedule was free after the surgery he was completing so they added me into that slot. For this reason the resident wheeled me down instead of patient transportation. My husband understands better than I do what each physician understands and is responsible for. He grew concerned that my internist hadn't been contacted to help manage my blood sugar during surgery. Of course the surgeon or anesthesiologist can do it, but not nearly with the skill of an internal medicine doctor. So Steve had my internist paged. He explained my situation and my internist met us outside the operating room and asked for my chart to write insulin and blood sugar management orders.

When I came out of surgery I was sent to the nephrology floor. The surgeon explained that a section of bowel slipped through a hole in my peritoneum. He further explained that it rarely occurs, however the wear of using the peritoneum as a filter in dialysis because the kidneys don't work, typically causes holes. Evidently I moved to just the right position to cause 10 inches of my bowel to slip through a hole in my peritoneum. The pinching of my bowel and my inability to get any food or water beyond that point caused the intense pain I was in.

Two months after the hernia operation, I had another incident. Although it wasn't a result of the transplant, the matter was complicated by my immunosuppression. My 11-year-old dog had a cancerous tumor that the vet said would be more risky to remove than to allow him to live as long as he could. As the tumor grew, it was difficult for Max to go up stairs. One day while trying to help him up the stairs, I accidentally pushed on his tumor and caused him pain. The only way a dog can say, "Don't do that," is to bite the hand that offended him. And so he quickly turned and bit my hand as he yelped. His bite broke the skin, even though it was not very painful. I quickly washed my hand with soap and allowed it to bleed under the flow of water, hoping to get rid of any bacteria.

Unfortunately, my hand began to swell. Once again we were headed to the ER. Doctors gave me IV antibiotics, but my hand continued to swell. It was my left hand that Max bit, and doctors were afraid that my wedding ring would cut off blood circulation in my hand and they asked if they could cut it off. I figured since it was April and our wedding anniversary was May 27th, a new wedding ring would be a perfect anniversary gift from my husband. The doctors tried to use wire snips but they didn't work. They used a small saw and in time they cut the ring. The rest of the story on getting a new wedding ring is that I didn't get one for another year and a half, during which I claimed to be unmarried.

It seems that all my emergency room visits are in the evening. The rest of the treatment was to give me two more IV bags of antibiotics. Doctors threatened to admit me but I explained that I had to be home by six the following morning in order to see my son off to school for a field trip and he needed a bag lunch. I also had a speaking engagement that evening. Therefore, rather than admit me to the hospital, they moved me to an extended stay room just off the emergency room. The plan was that the nurses had enough time to administer the IV antibiotics, as long as they wasted no time, for me to get home and meet my schedule. Since I was the person with so much to lose if my treatment wasn't finished as planned, I didn't sleep the balance of the night. I would nap between bags and as soon as one got close to empty, I pushed the nurses call light to change the bag.

With not a moment to spare, I got home in time to pack my son's lunch and see him and my husband off to school and work. I showered and left for work myself, right behind them. The speaking engagement that I had that evening was for NABAS Scholarship Fund. I was the treasurer of the Scholarship Fund and we were presenting several scholarships at the organization's annual fund raiser held at Cobo Hall in Detroit. This particular scholarship dinner was important to me because the guest speaker was the president of Lear Corporation. The student I was presenting a scholarship to had worked a summer internship at Lear, in fact, she worked with one of my own college roommates. I knew my roommate would attend the dinner and I wanted to make special mention of her mentorship and that she had been my roommate. Thanks to managing the doctors, my mission was accomplished.

The Future of Lewis Metal Stamping

While I managed to move the business while on dialysis, and the kidney transplant certainly made me feel like a new woman, I had to think very seriously about my ongoing responsibilities and abilities. Although I felt like I was on the road to recovery and would likely be as good as new, I had to objectively consider other facts. My company was small, and even though I was able to grow it some, I wasn't able to get it to a critical mass that could weather the brewing stormy economy that eventually made its way. All my contemplation seemed to point to one crucial question: Do I preserve my father's legacy or do I secure my son's future?

Although the thought of closing my father's business seemed to add a data point to the statistic of second generation businesses failing, and it seemed to be disrespectful to his memory, a step backwards in black business progress, not to mention that it pierced my heart, the decision seemed clear—preserve my son's future.

It took me months, years of working for colleagues to convince myself that closing the business didn't kill my father's legacy. In fact I know that if he were in the same predicament, he too would have chosen my future; that neither the buildings nor the business itself were my dad. All that he taught me, provided for me and protected me from is who my father was.

I first tried to sell the business or to relent to a 51-49

deal if I could work one out. Those interested in that kind of deal seemed to be a familiar shade of sleazy, either making me ultimately liable for a business they were in control of, or they wanted something for nothing. I couldn't bring myself to take that route; it wasn't what my father taught me, nor was it what my mentor had confirmed as the right way to understand business. Whatever I did, I needed to protect my mother personally from any financial liability associated with the business. I had already negotiated with the bank to release her personal guarantee after the loan had been paid down to a certain level, and it was below that level and I received verification that she was taken off of the loan. To remove her from personal liability as owner of the buildings that we operated in, we formed an LLC that received the rent payments and listed the LLC as loss payee on the business insurance.

Ultimately, I decided that closing the business was best. I notified my employees on the last working day of 2001 that I would cease operations. While this was a difficult Christmas present, it was probably the best time for me to pay them for a week of vacation to look for another job. Separating people from their means of feeding their family is never an easy thing to do—whether it was laying someone off or firing them. My father used to tell me that if ever I am happy separating someone from their job, something must be wrong with me. Certainly closing the business was even more hurtful.

My plant manager and I were the only two remaining as we turned as much raw material into sales as we could. We managed to supply customers and ship tools in time that there were no interruptions in product supply at the customer plants. When all was done, my business mentor, by this time also my friend, employed both my former plant manager and me at his Michigan operation.

Another Transplant

After the kidney transplant, doctors told me that the best thing to preserve my kidney would be a pancreas transplant. A pancreas transplant would mean that my blood sugar would be normal. The pancreas transplant would not only preserve my new kidney but stop the progression of other long term complications of diabetes like retinopathy or neuropathy. The pancreas is a more delicate organ than the kidney. Therefore the transplant is more difficult. I had been diabetic for 32 years; since I was seven years old. The appealing part of the prospect of a pancreas transplant was that I wouldn't have the aggravation of low and high blood sugars, nor would I have such an involved maintenance schedule in order to remain healthy. I would have more time to care for my son and to concentrate on re-establishing my career without the burden of managing diabetes. That prospect would have been exciting, except I wouldn't allow myself to look across the river and imagine what life would be like with a functioning pancreas. I was afraid of setting myself up for disappointment. I returned to the transplant team and was completely re-evaluated like a brand new transplant patient. I was officially listed on the pancreas transplant list, but I wouldn't let myself think about it too often nor would I sit and imagine what it would be like.

At the end of May, I was working at my mentor's company

on a pricing proposal that needed to be emailed in minutes, while also mentally preparing for a conference call scheduled to begin in five minutes. I was paged. The only reason I carried the pager was for transplant, but I of course used it for other things. I looked at the number and told myself that I would return the call later. The rules of transplant are that you have exactly one hour to respond otherwise they will go to the next person in line on the transplant list. It was transplant that paged and the nurse was growing frustrated. Once again, my high school friend Richard stepped in when the nurse asked him, "Do you know where she is?" I had emailed Richard with my work email and phone number. He called and said, "Hey, what's wrong with you, don't you want a pancreas?" I thought he was kidding and I tried to brush him off of the phone. He said, "No, really, we have a pancreas for you, but you have to talk to the nurse now!"

Needless to say, I responded to the page and called the transplant coordinator. And so the next morning, May 30th, 2002 at 7 a.m., I received the pancreas. To my amazement, my little brother drove in from Chicago to see me before surgery. According to my husband's search of public records and funerals in Michigan we believe it was the pancreas of a young woman who died tragically in a car accident. Many times I think of her family and how courageously they made the decision to donate her organs. My life is extended and I'm able to raise my precious son, who was then an 11-year-old, and needed me then more than ever to start Middle School.

When my grandmother came to visit me in the hospital, I reminded her of what Granddaddy promised me as a little girl when I was first diagnosed diabetic. He said that we would pray it [diabetes] away. Somehow, when he said it, I imagined that one day I would magically wake up and not need to take insulin anymore. I think often when we pray for God to bless us; we think in simple terms and believe that everything will be done with divine intervention. Certainly there are examples of those kinds of medical miracles—like the child who survived a plane crash when everyone else aboard was killed. While God certainly has that kind of power, He is also complex. He uses others to carry out blessings, even to the point that we believe that the powers to heal are our own. In the medical profession it is known as having a God Complex. God doesn't always answer prayers by supernaturally changing situations. Instead He creates opportunities for our desires to be realized.

I think the same is true for my grandfather's statement. God didn't wake me up one morning to discover that I was no longer diabetic. He created an opportunity for me to have a kidney transplant, which is why doctors would even consider a pancreas transplant, and the pancreas transplant ended my insulin dependence. Granddaddy was right; he prayed it away.

I had been diabetic since I was seven years old. To all of a sudden have what I referred to as an automatic pancreas was something to get used to. So many people, myself included, thought that a pancreas transplant would be so liberating—I would be free from taking insulin shots, free to eat what I wanted, etc. Instead, I could feel my blood sugar raising and dropping. The first thing that I noticed was that my morning blood sugar levels always felt like I was having a low blood sugar reaction. So I would always eat as soon as I woke up. Doctors explained that my new pancreas was surgically connected directly to my large intestine. This sent insulin straight to my blood stream rather than through my liver as the insulin was routed with my native pancreas. Because the insulin goes directly into the blood stream and doesn't receive some glucose from my liver, my morning blood sugars are lower than the normal range. The doctors suggested that I do nothing. My hypoglycemic symptoms would adjust to what is now my new normal blood sugar. It took a while, but I refrained from eating immediately after getting out of bed. Sure enough my morning fasting blood sugar normalized at about 77 and I no longer had hypoglycemic symptoms.

I tested my new automatic pancreas. After I ate a piece of chocolate or after a heavy meal I would test my blood sugar to see if it had gone up to 300 like it used to do. It consistently measured at or about 200, which is normal for after eating a heavy meal. As time went on, my husband remarked on how my skin looked better and that my feet were no longer cold. The dentist remarked how much healthier my gums were. The pancreas transplant really had improved my overall health.

❀ ❀ ❀

Chapter Seven

Victory Lap

A Test of Endurance and Proof that He Lives!

$\mathcal{T}$he pancreas transplant meant going back to square one as far as transplant monitoring is concerned. I had to go back to maintaining my logs of weight, blood pressure, blood sugar, and temperature several times a day. Process is the key for successful outcomes in these situations. As soon as you become complacent and believe that you are cured, anything can go wrong. Just four months after my pancreas transplant, I felt like I was coming down with a cold. I managed to get my son off to school, and my mother came over to see how she could help. As called for in my daily monitoring of my systems, I took my temperature and it was 99. I began to feel worse, I again took my temperature and it read 101. My husband was insistent that we call the U of M Transplant Center. The nurses reminded me that the protocol was to come to the ER. So off to the ER we went, like we had done so many times before.

When I arrived at the ER, they were expecting me. I waited briefly in a private waiting area and then was seen by the triage nurse. I've come to expect the royal treatment that transplant patients get because of our immunosuppressed status. They quickly drew blood and expected that I was rejecting one of the organs. But test results showed that neither of my organs were being rejected. I was obviously ill from something. I then remembered that it was the last day of the incubation period from my son's chicken pox vaccination. The chicken pox vaccine is a live virus and is dangerous for immunosuppressed patients. I had the option of not getting him vaccinated despite school rules, but I decided to. The pediatrician told me to make sure we continued to do lots of hand washing, not to kiss on the mouth, and that I should abstain from washing his clothes for 60 days. I remember marking on the calendar when that 60 day incubation period would end. It happened that it was on my aunt's birthday, so it would be easy to remember. Well, it also happens that we were in the ER on my aunt's birthday. I mentioned to the nurse to check for the chicken pox virus, that perhaps I hadn't escaped the virus despite all my precautions. She tested and assured me that it wasn't chicken pox. I was obviously ill, but they couldn't find a cause for it. They admitted me in order to do more extensive testing.

This part of my hospital stay gets very foggy and most of what I know was told to me by my husband, mother, son, cousin and friends. Again, because of the royal treatment I get by being immunosuppressed, and also because they couldn't identify what was wrong with me, I was admitted into a private room. Within two days my condition worsened to an almost coma. According to my mother, husband and girlfriend, I told them that doctors had released me and that they should come and get me. None of this was true. In fact doctors were confused as to what could be causing my illness. My speech was slurred beyond comprehension; I had no motor control of my hands and couldn't turn over in bed. I was light sensitive. My mother told me that the drapes were drawn, but the crack of sunlight which came between them gave me a headache; so she stood between me and the crack of sunlight coming through the window – work only a mom would think of doing.

Steve was afraid that he might lose his wife, and Stevie kept asking him if Mommy was going to die. Steve knew he had to be honest with his 12-year-old, but he didn't know himself. One day while running between Beverly Hills and Ann Arbor—taking my son to school and going to the hospital (about a 40 mile drive) Steve was on his cell phone with our friend, and according to her, he wasn't making sense. She asked him to pull over to the side of the road. She called another friend of ours, our pastor, who came to pick him up and drove him to the hospital. Although they don't talk much about that incident, I am sure the pastor helped to calm Steve spiritually.

Because the doctors at the hospital had to tell him only what they knew, Steve needed a friend with the medical understanding to explain to him what was likely to occur. We had befriended a family from Stevie's school whose sons were friends of Stevie's. Both parents are physicians, and Steve asked the boy's dad to drive with him to visit me and explain whether he (our doctor friend) thought I would live. I have no recollection of our doctor friend visiting, as well as several others who said they visited. Steve says he examined me and began teaching the residents to look at my neurological signs. It was clear that I had some neurological deficits. In answer to Steve's question, all he could say is that we would know in 48 hours whether I would make it.

I was seen by infectious disease doctors who ordered a spinal tap. I was tested at U of M and a second blood sample was flown to the Center for Disease Control in Atlanta, and they confirmed that I had the West Nile virus. There is no treatment for the West Nile virus. The body either fights the virus off or it overtakes the body. My chances of fighting it off were slim because of the immunosuppressant drugs I was taking. But because my transplant doctors were right there and monitoring my treatment, they were able to take me off of the anti-rejection drugs for a while so that my body could fight the virus. Everyone, except me because I was not lucid, held their breath. In addition to the fear that my immune system couldn't fight the virus, they were also afraid that suspending my anti-rejection drugs would cause my immune system to fight my transplanted organs. As God would have it, my body fought the West Nile virus while God protected my transplanted organs.

Indeed, my body began to fight the virus. But my near month long battle left me weak and not able to walk or talk. Because I had no memory of the time I spent in the hospital with West Nile, to me it seemed as if I was in a coma and then came out of it. My earliest memory of coming out of the coma from West Nile is waking up one morning feeling sweaty and dirty. I realized that I was in a hospital and somehow that didn't startle me. It was as if I knew that part. I heard workmen banging in the hallway and the sound of power saws. For some reason, I believed that they were tearing down a movie set that was staged so that my cousin's 25th wedding anniversary party guests could watch me on a hidden camera while I was in the hospital. Now that I've had time to analyze my initial thoughts when coming out of the coma, I think that prior to going to the hospital I was looking forward to my cousin's party and preparing mental notes to congratulate them publicly at the event. The party was still on my mind while I took a vacation from reality, and returned when I returned to reality.

A nurse came in to check my IV and I asked her if she was a real nurse or an actress. She explained that she was indeed a nurse. So I concluded that perhaps I really was in a hospital and these were not actors on a set. I also resolved in my mind that it would be boring for my cousin's guests to watch me on hidden camera as entertainment for the party.

Later in the evening, or one evening—time is difficult to determine—I recall waking up and trying to walk to the bathroom myself. I fell and lost my bowels all over the bathroom. A nurse's aide found me in the bathroom. She checked to see if I was ok and then ran for the nurse. They came back seconds later and cleaned me up and got me back to bed. While the nurse's aide cleaned the bathroom, I apologized to both of them. The nurse explained to me that it was no problem, and it is imperative that I get help walking anywhere. She explained that I had been in the bed for a long time and was weak. She told me that she didn't mind helping me to the bathroom whenever I needed to go. I guess I had no idea that I wasn't able to walk unassisted.

I lost 30 pounds while in the hospital. I was very weak physically and my speech was impaired. Doctors were concerned about my ability to eat, because the muscles in my mouth were not working properly; chewing was as big of a chore as speaking. My doctors threatened to put a feeding tube in my nose if I wasn't able to regain some of the weight. After my last experience with an NG tube, that was plenty motivation for me.

Upon discharge from the hospital, the doctor gave me a prescription for Vicodin, for pain relief. When the doctor left, I asked Steve why he gave it to me. When I left the hospital, I was very weak and incredibly dizzy, so I couldn't imagine taking Vicodin because it would make me even dizzier. Steve told me that I had been complaining about pain. Even then, I had no recollection of pain. I also have no recollection of light sensitivity as my mother described.

I finally went home. And with me came a wheelchair, a walker, a shower seat and a bedside commode—which I refused to use. I used my walker to get to the bathroom and back. It felt so good to be home. The first thing that I had to do was to take a shower to get that institutional smell off of me.

No doubt I hadn't had anything more than a bedside wash up for a month. So my husband and nurse friend Karon, got me upstairs, ran some bath water and sat me in the tub. As hard as that was for them to do, lifting me out soaked and wet was even more difficult. The effects of fighting West Nile left me too weak to walk so I used a wheelchair. It left me with a speech impediment that made it difficult for people to understand me or what I wanted. I was dizzy; laying down stopped the room from spinning. As soon as I arrived home, before the home therapists could get started, friends of ours began working with me on speech therapy and the occupational therapy of getting around the house with limited balance and mobility. Steve's childhood friend Greg went through the house recommending items that would help me to get around the house. We had a colonial with a stairway with a 90 degree turn and landing to complete the ascent to the next level. Greg recommended that we put a chair on the landing so that I could rest between flights of stairs. He was absolutely right. I was so tired half way up that I needed to take a rest. It's hard to imagine that the concentration and physical exertion of climbing the steps would be so tiring, but it was.

Thea, my college roommate and now a Speech Pathologist, came promptly with words for me to practice pronouncing and passages for me to read aloud and to practice where to pause and take a breath. Thea amazed me at how efficiently she worked. Her mother is a stroke survivor and had trouble with memory recall. So the homework she gave me was to make three lists each day: one list of all the people who came to visit, another list of the things I did during the day, and finally a list of what I had to do tomorrow. I had no idea until this point that I didn't have strength enough to hold a pen and write. So this exercise helped me gain strength enough to write. Thea instructed me to call her mother everyday at 1 p.m. with that list. Her mother would then relay the message to Thea. It took me several weeks to understand that Thea had complicated therapy going on with two patients—me and her mother. I then felt obligated to call—I couldn't miss, I couldn't mess up Mama Covington's therapy!

Within a week of getting home, I received speech, physical and occupational home therapy. As a part of my occupational therapy, I straightened up my kitchen and cooked meals that didn't require that I stand for long periods of time. While picking up the kitchen, I found a portable radio on the book shelf. I took it down and put it on the table for someone to take it upstairs later. I didn't recognize the radio, but I figured it didn't belong in the kitchen. My son came downstairs and asked me "Is Jackie coming over?" Jackie is my business colleague and my girlfriend who bought the $400 make-up brushes at the spa. We often did things together because our kids were the same age. I answered Stevie, "No, why do you ask?" Stevie said "Because that's her radio." I asked why it was here. Stevie asked me, "Don't you remember? The doctors said that a radio would be good to lie near your head in the hospital to try to arouse you. Jackie brought her radio." I put my head in my hands to cry. I knew that I didn't meet her by chance; that God placed her in my life for that reason and many more.

Rehabilitation continues to be a slow process. As time progresses, much of what I recall is feeling like I had a cold when I left for the emergency room, and then the rehabilitation when I got home. There aren't many days that I go without considering this West Nile experience. It is a real mystery for me and primarily a series of stories from friends and family.

At home, I had to figure out how I would maneuver around the house and begin to resume my duties as a wife and mother, which took longer than I imagined. My occupational therapist worked with me on ways to begin getting back to working around the house. She helped me think of new ways to endure standing and preparing dinner. To make beef stew in my roaster, I would season the beef and place it in the roaster with a little water. I would rest a few minutes and then balance on my walker while peeling potatoes. Peeling the potatoes was the most difficult task. My dexterity was terrible and my strength was barely enough to cut the potato with the knife. I was dizzy, which made it difficult to stand for a long time. My coordination was non-existent. Peeling potatoes looked more like whittling wood. After a break, I would add carrots and onions, put it on low heat and let it slow cook.

Another work out was to practice typing. I was used to typing more than 40 words per minute. I soon found that my impaired dexterity slowed my speed dramatically. Not only was my dexterity slow, but because I lost some control of my eye muscles, focusing my eyes on the screen was difficult to do. I did occupational therapy exercises where I followed the square shape of a window in the room, the doorway, then smaller objects like tables and other furniture, then smaller square objects like boxes or bricks. This was to gain better control of my eye muscles and focus. I could remember the keyboard, but couldn't coordinate my fingers to type the words in the fluid motion I was used to. With practice, I improved. The typing exercise culminated in a Christmas letter that I sent to friends and family

While I was working on the computer, I remembered that I was about to pay bills when I went to the hospital. Knowing that my husband stepped in while I was away, I decided to see where things stood. Steve said that he paid "some." Sure enough when I looked at our checking account and the balance of outstanding bills, I guess my husband paid what he felt was important. Our house note was nearly 60 days old, however the cable bill had been paid so many times that it didn't need to be paid for the next couple of months. I asked my husband what the plan was– did he intend to ask the new owners of the house if he could live in the backyard and run an extension cord to be able to watch his cable TV?

Nearly two years after my illness, I recalled my husband saying that he brought the digital video camera to the hospital for me to see one of Stevie's school soccer games. I decided to get the camera and insert the digital card into the computer to see the footage. It was there, but to my surprise and amazement, there were also pictures of me in the hospital during West Nile. It was proof that these stories were true.

Not that I doubted their validity, but it was a picture of what I couldn't imagine.

There were four still pictures: two of friends of mine who visited, one of me and a nurse listening to my lungs, and another of my mother and friends of ours looking at me. What amazed me was that my eyes were open and I was smiling— not at the camera, but at my mother and friends. Somehow through all the stories I imagined myself as being in a coma. But the picture proved that wasn't so. I don't remember, but my eyes were open.

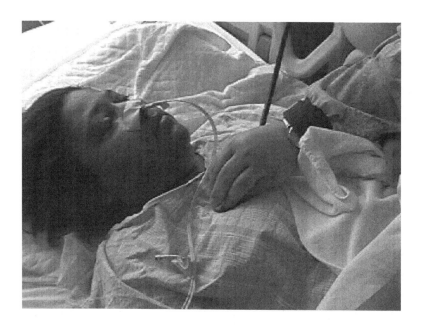

✿ ✿ ✿

Epilogue

In my private devotion with God, I reflected on my two transplants and how only through God's grace could all of this miraculous healing be possible. As I further reflected upon my life, I realized that as organized as I like to think I am, there couldn't have been a better, more efficient way of making me the person I had become. My unending praise came from not just what God had done for me in the last two years, but how my steps were ordered in college, being trained by my father and ultimately becoming CEO of his business. Yes, as I reflected on my near 40 years of life, I had lived a fuller life than most live in 80 years of life. It was then that I thanked God and told Him that if He never blessed me again, I had received more than my share of blessings. As if the pool of blessings that God bestowed is some sort of zero sum apportionment, I felt I had received more than my allotment. And for that I was thankful and ready to die whenever God called me home.

When I look back on my life, I am more blessed than most. I was born to two incredible parents who taught me that I could be whoever I wanted to be as long as I worked hard at it, despite diabetes. They provided me with a stellar education both at college and at Lewis Metal Stamping. Little did I know that my father was preparing me to one day run the business on my own—and that I did for eight years. I've married a wonderful husband who has helped me (in sickness and in health) raise a successful son. What more is there?

In fact, I believe the highs and lows of my life have taught me lots. For instance, I believe that my juvenile diabetes has taught me to aggressively pursue my desires. At 7 I had to be attuned with my body in order to recognize potentially dangerous symptoms. Therefore I have grown up very aware of my environment and I also recognized that it would take a little extra work for me to complete what most have to do because I have to also maintain my health. But if you grow up with the mantra, "it will take a little more work for me and so I need to start early," then it is natural to just get the work done and not make excuses or whine about the workload. Besides that, I believe I learned from the ultimate multi-tasker, my mother. I believe the ability to handle activities that others thought were restrictive, tedious or just plain difficult came easier to me because I had to manage my diabetes.

Sometimes we fall into the trap of looking at life as teenagers do—what matters is what happened most recently. And most recently I have been ill and in hospitals. The illnesses that occurred in a matter of three years have given me a greater understanding of who my parents and grandparents taught me to trust. When I imagine what could have happened so many times or worse yet, things that might not have happened, I say thank you Jesus. My transplants still feel like medical miracles. I don't care how close siblings are; perhaps the greatest test of a sibling's love is whether they would donate an organ to save your life. There are actually two tests—one is the medical test to see if you are medically capable, and the second is a test of Christian love—an unconditional love. I am one of few who knows that my brother unequivocally loves me. What more could I want?

In review of all that has happened to me in my life, all the hospitalizations and all the surgeries, I don't recall being afraid. I've had a lot to fear. But I remember very clearly sitting in the surgical waiting room for my brother's surgery to be near complete before they took me back to prepare to receive his kidney. I wasn't worried. It was 2:30 in the afternoon and I was happy that I would be receiving anesthesia soon to distract me from being hungry. Again, when my husband walked with me on the stretcher going to the operating room to receive the pancreas, we were busy asking the nurse if I would be well enough in a month to go white water rafting. My brother drove in from Chicago, and he was a wonderful sight to see just before they wheeled me into the operating room. Was my faith so strong that worry wasn't in the equation?

I did in fact have faith that my God wouldn't bring me to so much and not bring me through it. But as I questioned my faith during those critical times, I know that there was something more working. So much could have gone wrong. My brother, a mere 32-year-old kid, could have lost his life trying to save mine. Still diabetic during the kidney transplant, my blood sugar could have dropped or soared causing other medical and surgical problems. What if the kidney didn't function in my body? What if after the gift of life from the donor family, the pancreas didn't work? What if I bled to death? All those things that could go wrong during surgery that you read about – what if any one of those things occurred? I did have faith in my transplant team, but most especially in God that He would guide the surgeons' minds, hands and hearts.

To think that I was diagnosed diabetic at the age of seven and took insulin shots for 32 years, and then I walked into the hospital one afternoon and after the next morning's surgery, I never took insulin again – it's amazing. To show how quickly we adapt to change, I sometimes wonder if I could give myself a shot now. But perhaps the most spiritual of the journeys that I have been on in my life is that of West Nile Encephalitis. All I can recall of my West Nile journey is the ER visit and what my family and friends told me. It is amazing that I cannot recall almost a month of time in the hospital. Understanding as I do from my husband's accounts, my situation was very grave. Whenever I try to discuss with my husband the details of what was going on while I was sick with West Nile, his eyes glass over and his comments are short. When I talk to other friends and family, their conversations are rather short as well. Even doctors and nurses, when I returned for follow-up visits or blood tests, stop and say to me that they are so pleased to see me doing well, because I was so sick before. I can only gather from this that I was nearer to death than I ever imagined.

When I talk about the time that I don't remember and was in the hospital with West Nile, I refer to it as when I was on vacation. I call it a vacation because I don't remember all of the pain and medical procedures that I went through. And I couldn't have been worried, because I don't remember what was going on. The only way I can describe this experience is to borrow the words the poet Mary Stevenson uses in her poem Footprints in the Sand,

> *"My son, my precious child,*
> *I love you and I would never leave you.*
> *During your times of trial and suffering,*
> *when you see only one set of footprints,*
> *it was then that I carried you."*

Pressing that thought further, I asked myself, why would God send me through such a serious health battle? What had I done to deserve not only this serious brush with death, but two transplants before it, all in three years? I searched for reasons, and as with everyone, I could come up with a list of reasons that God could punish me. But as I thought up this list, I prayed and asked God for forgiveness for these things all over again. I thought about how people reacted when I asked them what went on when I was in the hospital with West Nile. I recalled that my son, while not an adult, was 11 years old and could recount what happened, never said much at all. My husband, if in a group, let others answer instead of him. My mother in quiet moments alone told me the most, after which we usually cried. I believe that God was showing me that my stent with West Nile in fact had very little to do with me. It was something that my body went through, however God used me to demonstrate to others around me what He is capable of.

I have never before lost my memory and therefore not to remember what happened for a month in the hospital seemed unreal. My husband told me of all the hospital visitors; of my college roommate who visited early to make sure I was cleaned up by the time my mother came to the hospital, of church congregations that prayed for my recovery, and of other close friends and family. Lots of people saw me and what happened to me. Even medical professionals at the hospital and at clinics that I went to for tests after I went home were able to see how very gravely ill I was and how God brought me through it. That is why I believe the victory and blessing of surviving and overcoming the test, trials and tribulations of my life, although it happened to me, were not just for me. I believe it was for others to witness and to grow in faith.

As I understood that God used me, I remembered back to when Granddaddy was diagnosed a second time with lung cancer and how I wanted God to use me in that situation. Here it was some 20 years later, and God had used me. He probably has used me in other circumstances, but for certain, He used me during my West Nile illness. As Christians, we often think that everything that happens to us is about us. West Nile was so not about me, but about teaching those who witnessed God's power and might. Understanding where I've been and the preparation that I've received from God, my parents, my schools, my work experiences and the people around me, who better could God have chosen to demonstrate his blessed assurance?

❀ ❀ ❀

About The Author

In *Blessed Assurance*: Success Despite the Odds, Jacquie Lewis-Kemp illustrates God's grace through her journey at age 7 with juvenile diabetes, through the excitement and disappointment of working for her father's automotive manufacturing company from Production Control Manager to CEO, and finally through her trials of long term complications of diabetes. Her's is a story of discipline and of God's blessed assurance.

Jacquie Lewis-Kemp still resides in Michigan with her husband and son, dog Lizzy and cats Picasso and Maya. She is an active member of Hope United Methodist Church, participating in the United Methodist Women and Church & Society ministries. Jacquie no longer works in the automotive supplier industry and is now an aspiring author with lots of book ideas. She keeps her analytical skills sharp by working with friends on business plans and other business projects.

In 2004, Jean Lewis, Jacquie's mom, suffered a stroke and was pronounced brain dead. Having witnessed firsthand the life restoration of transplant, Jeff and Jacquie carried out their mother's wish to donate her organs. Jean's gift of life gave sight to two and a life saving liver to a third. Spiritually, Jeff and Jacquie understand that once God calls the spirit home, the body is merely the remaining shell that the spirit inhabited while on earth. Organ donation is a way of restoring physical health and blessing someone's walk on this earth after a loved one has been called home.

At the time of this printing, it has been nine years since the kidney transplant and seven years since the pancreas transplant. Praise God from whom all blessings flow!

To order additional copies of *Blessed Assurance* visit our website www.zoelifepub.com. On the website you will also find information about other books by Zoë Life Publishing destined to change the world one life at a time through the power of the written word.

A bulk discount is available when purchasing large quantities for retail or ministry purposes.

Contact Outreach at Zoë Life Publishing:

Zoë Life Publishing
P.O. Box 871066
Canton, MI 48187
(877) 841-3400
outreach@zoelifepub.com

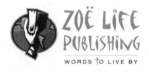